HISTORY C

C000146678

The definite guide
and deadliest epidemics and pandemics that
changed our world.

From the Roman Empire to the Modern Era

DAVID ANVERSA

2020 © David Anversa

This is the story of the largest epidemics and pandemics that have changed our world.
Millions of people have died, empires have fallen, and generations have been annihilated. David Anversa, in collaboration with a medic specializing in infectious diseases, traces the incredible stories of the most serious and terrible epidemics and pandemics that afflicted humanity from a medical, social, and economic point of view. We will start from the plagues that afflicted the Roman Empire and Ancient Greeks up to the present day.

I hope you will like this book! If you like, leave a positive review with your impressions on the Amazon page.
I would be really grateful! Check my other books in the Author Page on Amazon, you will find them very interesting!

For any kind of request, clarification or advice, feel completely free to contact me at the following email address:
davidanversa.author@gmail.com
Thank you very much and happy reading

David Anversa

CONTENTS:

Brief History of Medicine and Introduction to Microorganisms

Medicine is a discipline that dates back to when man discerned the difference between ill-health and health. It can be defined as the study of the treatment of diseases and injuries. Different societies had their own ways of explaining and tackling diseases and injuries even before the coming of conventional medicine. Some communities believed that health was a gift from the gods, and their wrath caused the lack of it. Hippocrates is considered the Father of Medicine and the first physician in the world. He contributed to modern medicine in that he believed that there was a rational explanation and physical cause of illness. Hippocrates lived around 400 BC, and needless to say, in that period, people did not have much knowledge concerning medicine. He contributed so much in the field of epidemiology, and some of his discoveries are utilized in modern medicine. The Chinese used herbal remedies and acupuncture starting 2200 years ago. These remedies are still used by people who prefer traditional medicine to conventional medicine. Moreover, the Chinese contributed to the field of surgery. The Babylonians are people who cannot be forgotten when talking about the history of medicine. They have early medicine texts which date back to the first half of the second millennium BCE. They believed that two kinds of people were responsible for the health of the society; the priest, also known as the exorcist and the physician. They healed illnesses such as depression, troubles with ears, and epilepsy. Indians also contributed significantly to medicine, especially in surgery. They helped people understand that health is not only physical well-being but also the mental and spiritual well-being of an individual. Have you ever heard of King Djoser, the chief of dentists and doctors? He was an Egyptian who contributed significantly to medicine. Egyptians came up with medical procedures such as mummification and other remedies in medicine. Medicine has evolved so much. Before Louis Pasteur came up with the germ theory, people knew very little to do with microorganisms and their disease-causing capacity. For the discovery of the germ theory, Louis Pasteur is known as the Father of Immunology. Today, people can not only identify disease-causing microorganisms but also tell their structure, differentiate one from the other and even tell when they mutate. By so doing, we can not only fight microorganisms but also get immunized so that the body can efficiently fight it off in case of an infection. We have also identified organisms that are helpful to the body, commonly referred to as commensals; this includes Escherichia coli found along the human digestive tract. Edward Jenner came up with the very first vaccine in the history of humankind. It was first tested on his wife. This knowledge is used almost everywhere in the world. Believe it or not, immunization prevents 2-3 million deaths annually, globally. Joseph Lister applied Pasteur's knowledge in his practice, and he pioneered antiseptic surgery, which is used up to date. Other pioneers in medicine include William Osler, the Father of Modern Medicine, who pioneered clinical bedside teaching of medical students, making the learning more practical. Florence Nightingale is the founder of nursing. Organ transplant is essential in treating organ failures in modern medicine. It was first carried out by Richard Lawler. He carried out the first successful kidney transplant. The tools and instruments that are used in the field of medicine and surgery have changed from basic tools to more sophisticated equipment. Traditional items include scissors, saws, and scalpels, which over the ages have become more refined. In the recent past, more surgeries have been carried out on delicate parts of the body, such as the brain and heart. There are also robotic surgeries that are very precise. At this time, we may think that a stethoscope is a fundamental part of the medical life, but before Rene Laennec invented the stethoscope in 1816, the physician had to place their ear near the patient's heart to hear the heartbeat. The stethoscope has evolved from the rod-like structure that Laennec invented to the efficient instrument that we know today. The first reliable mechanical ventilator was invented by Forrest Bird, and they are widely used in cardiopulmonary care. We can, therefore, say that medicine as a discipline has evolved and continues to develop due to the contributions of different people in different disciplines making medicine more efficient and reliable. Of all the things that exist, the microorganisms are the most interesting of them all. They are invisible to the naked eye, but their impact is enormous. For ages, man has been trying to explain the cause of disease. At times disease has been attributed to things such as the wrath of gods and other supernatural elements. It was not until Louis Pasteur developed the germ theory that we humans, started to appreciate the importance of microorganisms in our daily lives. Developments started occurring involving microorganisms, from the coining of the term cell by Robert Hooke to understanding their structure, multiplication, and the diseases they cause. Viruses are microorganisms that we encounter in our daily lives; for instance, the Flu is caused by viruses that affect the lungs and the upper respiratory tract. Other viruses include HIV, which causes AIDS, Epstein-Barr Virus, Varicella zoster, which causes Chickenpox, among others. A virus is a small microorganism that is unique in that it can only replicate in the cells of a living organism. When a virus is outside a living organism, it is essentially non-living as it cannot replicate or carry out any metabolic activity. Viruses can infect different kinds of living organisms ranging from bacteria (these viruses are known as bacteriophages), plants, animals, and most importantly, they can infect human beings. Some viruses cause zoonotic diseases, which can be transferred from animals to man. There are different kinds of viruses, but all of them have one thing in common; they use the living cell's machinery to replicate and affect the body. There are different kinds of viruses. There are enveloped and non-enveloped viruses. Enveloped viruses have an outer viral layer that protects its inner structure and genetic composition while un-enveloped viruses lack the outer viral layer. Coronavirus is an example of an enveloped virus, while poliovirus is un-enveloped. The genetic material of viruses can be DNA: single-stranded or double-stranded or RNA: single-stranded or rarely, double-stranded. Bacteria are maybe the most well-known microorganisms. They live in both man and animals and can be transmitted from animals to man. There are different types of viruses, such as gram-positive bacteria and gram-negative bacteria. There are Archaebacteria that exist in hostile environments such as hot springs and salt lakes. Eubacteria are found almost everywhere on earth. Gram-positive bacteria have a substance known as peptidoglycan, while gram-negative bacteria lack this substance. Bacteria can also be classified according to the shapes of their body. We have bacilli which are rod-shaped. An example of bacilli bacteria is Yersinia pestis that causes plague. Cocci (singular coccus) is another type of bacteria; the bacteria are spherical. They include Streptococcus pneumoniae. Spirilla (singular spirillum) are helical shaped bacteria. Campylobacter jejuni is a helical bacterium that causes campylobacteriosis. There are other types of bacteria, but these are the main types. Fungi are a group of microorganisms found on earth. Yeasts, rusts, smuts, mildews, molds, and mushrooms are examples of fungi. Fungi range from unicellular to multicellular organisms. There are fungi that are visible to the naked eye and those that are invisible. Fungi are fascinating in that some fungi cause diseases, while others are edible. It sounds incredible, right? Fungi cause oral thrush, candidiasis, among other conditions. On the other hand, some types of yeasts are used in the brewing of alcohol and to raise the dough. This shows that in as much as we are the drivers and controllers of the earth, microorganisms are essential and play an important role that no other organisms can. We have to consider them as we continue with our daily lives. We have to learn to preserve the useful microorganisms as well as combat the harmful ones.

Epidemics versus Pandemics and the differences

To understand the difference between these two commonly used and confusing terms, we will look into the epidemiology of infectious diseases. An infection is the entry, development, and establishment of an agent in the body of a host. The agent may be virulent, that is, it causes disease, or non-virulent, whereby it causes no disease. There are several gradients (levels) of infection, and they include: Sub-clinical (inapparent) infection Latent infection Colonization Manifest or clinical infection Subclinical infection is an infection that is nearly or completely asymptomatic. Therefore, the host of this microorganism is known as a carrier. In as much as the carrier is not affected by the agent, they may transmit it to other hosts who may show symptoms of the disease-causing agent. Chlamydia is a sexually transmitted infection that affects both men and women. In 75% of women and 50% of men, it is asymptomatic. This disease is therefore transmitted unknowingly. This is a good example of a subclinical infection that is asymptomatic. Latent infection can be described as an inactive or dormant infection. The disease-causing agent is not active in the sense that it does not replicate and may not cause symptoms. Many STD's undergo a latent period, whereby they are asymptomatic. During the latency period, the infection can still be transmitted from one individual to another, making the infections very dangerous. For instance, HIV infections are said to be latent when the virus is not replicating. The latent infection becomes active when the agent becomes active, replicates, and eventually causes symptoms. Colonization is very interesting in that there are bacteria on a body surface, for example, the intestines, mouth, skin, or the respiratory tract, but the bacteria do not affect the host. Staphylococcus aureus is a bacteria found on the skin and the upper respiratory tract. It is considered a member of the usual microbiota of the body. This kind of infection is known as colonization. Manifest or clinical infection is an infection that shows the clinical symptoms of a disease. The manifestation of infection may be local, for instance, an abscess, cellulitis, or systemic, like fever. Some diseases may have life-threatening manifestations, such as Septic Shock. A disease that is constantly present in a part of a region's population is referred to as *endemic*. The infection of this disease is maintained at the baseline level. For instance, malaria is endemic in Africa, and it contributes to 92% of WHO cases globally. An endemic disease may become an epidemic if the numbers of infected persons increase. An epidemic is defined as a widespread occurrence of an infectious disease at a particular time and in a particular community. Epidemics are caused by several factors that may be happening on the side of the host or of the agent. We can, therefore, group these factors as host factors or agent factors. Host factors affect the host and increase the chances of the host being infected by the disease-causing agent. They include: Increased susceptibility of the host, whereby a host that was previously immune to an agent of a disease, cannot be affected by the agent, hence by the disease. We have to remember that the susceptibility or resistance of a host is contributed to by several factors including genetic makeup, age, race, among other factors. Increased exposure of the host to the agent, increases the chances of the host being in contact with the disease-causing microorganisms, thus increasing the chances of infection. Agent factors are mechanisms that enhance the ability of an agent to infect a host. This includes: Increased virulence of the agent. Virulence is the ability of an agent to infect a host and cause disease. If the virulence goes up and the susceptibility remains the same, the host is more likely to contract the disease. An enhanced mode of transmission is another factor that causes epidemics. If the agents can be efficiently transmitted to the host, this means they can have access to the hosts more easily, thereby causing disease. An increase in the number of disease-causing microorganisms can cause an epidemic. An epidemic can affect the community enormously. It affects the economy greatly, and it may affect the beliefs of a society and its relations with each other. When an epidemic goes beyond a country's boundaries, it becomes a pandemic. For it to be considered a pandemic, it has to affect countries that are grouped in different regions by the World Health Organization (WHO). Pandemics that have affected the globe include; Spanish Flu, Cholera outbreak (1876), the Black Death (1345), HIV/AIDS (2005), and the most recent pandemic is the Coronavirus. Given that as a species, we have evolved, and we have more efficient ways of dealing with pandemics. I hope that we will not only contain coronavirus but also find vaccines and a cure so that we will save more lives, undergo less economic downfall, and come out stronger, wiser, and more experienced than we were before.

The Antonine Plague

During the reign of Emperor Marcus Aurelius, the Roman Empire was at the peak of its success. Their territory was vast and growing bigger with each passing victory in the battlefield, thanks to its hugely successful army. Trade was thriving more than ever before because the empire was not only taking part in the trade along the Silk Road but also had numerous trading ports. They had good leaders, and the most remarkable of them all was the wise, prudent, and powerful emperor, Marcus Aurelius. In short, the Roman Empire was the place to belong, and this filled the Romans with absolute pride. All was well until the Antonine plague, also known as the plague of Galen, struck the land. It was known that the emperor's surname was Antonius. The name, Plague of Galen, was because Galen was the physician who treated the majority of the people who suffered the plague. The disease was probably hitting Rome for the first time, and this was implied by the severity of the symptoms that the patients experienced. For quite some time, scientists tried to figure out which disease could have caused the Antonine Plague. All the symptoms pointed to smallpox, and it was unanimously agreed that one or two strains of the smallpox virus caused the epidemic. The Romans tried to explain the origin of this plague. Since the knowledge in medicine at that time was meager, all the Romans could do, was tell the pestilence using legends. In one of the myths, Lucius Verus, a leader of the army, opened a tomb in Seleucia, a city along the River Tigris. This act enraged the gods because it was a direct breaking of an oath against the pillage of the town. The gods released the plague as a sign of their burning wrath against the people. There was also another legend that a Roman soldier opened a golden casket in a temple of Athens in Babylon, releasing the plague. This was sacrilege and direct disrespect to the gods. The Romans were polytheists, but there were Christians who were also living in their land. The Christians were monotheists, and the polytheists believed that they did something that made the gods burn with rage against them. They blamed the plague on the

Christians and spotted them in every way possible. In a world that barely had any knowledge in science and was full of superstition, it is not surprising that these were the explanations they had. The Antonine Plague emerged in present-day China and spread along the Silk Road and to other parts of Asia. The Silk Road was a significant trade route that connected the East and the West. Its eastern end was in China while the western end was in Antioch. It was important not only because of the trade that was taking place but also in the cultural and religious interactions among the people who took part in the trade. It was called the Silk Road because the Chinese had conquered most towns along the route. The Roman Army attacked the town of Seleucia, intending to capture it. The people in Seleucia had been struck by a pestilence that left them vulnerable. It was also in this town that the soldiers came in contact with and contracted the Antonine Plague, and that was probably the reason they had the legend about the opening of the tomb in Seleucia. When the soldiers started presenting symptoms of the plague, it was only a matter of days that the disease began spreading, and people started dying. Galen documented the symptoms and course of this plague in his book, Methodus Medendi. The plague had signs that at first, it seemed like heavy flu. They were fever, coughing, and malaise- a general feeling of unwellness. Unlike the flu, the symptoms did not dwindle but rather became worse as the days went by. Galen recorded that one would have a pimple on the arms or legs. It would disappear then reappear on the torso, something that probably did not raise the alarm. On the fourth day, one would have exanthema, a rash that would get worse by the day. Imagine having pustules throughout the body, and the patients would have so much trouble while lying down or even dressing up because the pustules were not only painful but also itchy. The pustules were filled with pus and had a little depression in the middle, and they were not a pretty sight. After several days, scabs would form off the pimples. The scab tissue would then fall off, leaving pits and spots. Modern scientists have concluded that the disease was smallpox. The scientific names of the two strains of the smallpox virus are Variola major and Variola minor. Variola is a Latin name that means "spotted." This name may be referring to the spots that the patients retained after the scabs had fallen off. The patients had a sore and painful throat. They also had a constant feeling of thirst. They had headaches, muscle aches, and confusion. The monstrosity was very contagious, and it spread like a bushfire throughout Rome. From the army barracks to homes, palaces, temples, and the ports of trade, the contagion spread fast. The cities of Rome were densely populated, and this accelerated the spread of the illness. The people who were not already infected knew that it was only a matter of time until they could be infected by the disease. We know today that smallpox is mainly spread through bodily fluids. Therefore, it was spread via sputum while the patients were talking or coughing. At times the pustules would break, and those who came into contact with the fluid got infected. The disease was also spread by sharing beddings, clothing, and utensils. After presenting with symptoms, patients died after 2-3 weeks. This made the people feel as if the phantom of death was hovering over their heads and could strike at any time. Panic-stricken, the people started fleeing Rome, and Galen, the physician, fled and only came back after much persuasion by the leaders, including the emperor himself. We can only imagine how many others had fled the Empire. The disease was affecting all; the weak and poor, young and old, leader or civilian, farmer or trader. The Roman army was carrying out two military expeditions which promoted the spread of the disease. The first one, in which Marcus Aurelius took part, was the Parthia's war in Mesopotamia. The other one took part in Northern Italy in Pannonia and Noricum. The episodes were characterized by battles where soldiers came in contact with each other. The soldiers also dwelled in congested, dirty, and damp camps, which made it easy for the disease to propagate and spread. During these wars, the soldiers looted and carried treasure from the conquered land. The treasures were the fomites that carried the disease-causing microorganisms to Rome. The Antonine Plague took away so many lives. Each day, about 2000 people died in Rome. It decimated the population of Rome. The Roman army had 28 legions, which had a total of about 150,000 troops. The members were healthy foot-soldiers, seasoned horsemen, powerful commanders, with experienced physicians to take care of the soldiers. The army was the pride of the Roman people. Members of the military were well-disciplined, as well as victorious in their quests. The soldiers contracted the disease from their fellow soldiers and spread it on. The sick soldiers were weak and were distressed because they could no longer fight. Like everyone else, they were disillusioned because they knew that their only hope to escape the misery of this monstrosity was death. In an attempt to restore the dwindling glory of the army, Marcus Aurelius increased the rate of conscription. This may sound like a solution, but then let us not forget that the plague had also stricken the civilians. They were frail and untrained; most of them were grieving the loss of their loved ones or taking care of their terribly sick relatives. As they say, misfortunes never come singly, and without a well-functioning army, the people were vulnerable to external attacks. Some German tribes took advantage of this situation and attacked some parts of Rome and occupied the territory. It's not easy to experience the loss of family members, colleagues, age-mates, and leaders all at the same time. The people were exhausted emotionally, as they were always grieving and anxious. The people dreaded contracting the pestilence because they knew that they would end up dead. The plague weakened the empire in almost all sectors. The people could not take part in trading as they were either taking care of sick family members or were too scared to contract the disease while trading. Commodities were scarce, and prices rose. Therefore, only wealthy merchants could carry on with the trade. Some of the traders died, and their numbers drastically reduced. Farmers were significantly affected by this monstrosity; they were weak and could not till the land, sow seeds, weed, or even harvest. This impacted the shortage of food throughout the empire. The farmers could no longer produce cotton, which was an essential commodity for export; this weakened the economy. The craftsmen could no longer make pieces of art to adorn cities, temples, streets, homes, or for trade. Those who used to mine precious stones could no longer do that. The number of taxpayers went down as people died during the plague. The impoverished citizens could not contribute tax in the same measure as when they were healthy. Less tax meant meager wages for those who were working and even fewer provisions to the weakened nation if there were any. Physicians and caretakers also, at times, got the plague and died. No one was safe. The Antonine Plague was said to have been caused by the Christians who were dwelling in Rome. The polytheists accused them of committing sacrilege, thus enraging the gods. The Christians were persecuted and spited by the polytheists. They were maltreated more than ever before. Contrary to the expectations, the Christians showed utter compassion and love to the polytheists. They responded to blame, with kindness, and hatred, with love. They took care of the ill and suffering, whether they were Christians or not. They never blamed the polytheists for persecuting them but took care of them without complaining. This astounded the polytheists as this was contrary to the teachings of the Polytheistic religion. The Christian faith gave the polytheists a glimmer of hope; it taught about life after death. This life would be without suffering or want of any kind. Some polytheists converted to Christianity; this way, they died more peacefully, expecting something better than all the agony they had experienced. The Antonine Plague, therefore, caused a change in religion in Rome. Some Christians contracted the disease while attending to sick people. Most of these Christians died. They died believing that they were serving a good cause. In as much as the plague killed many people, some recovered from the disease and became resistant to it. This is known as acquired immunity. These people were urged to help and take care of those who were ailing because they were immune to the disease. The Antonine Plague impacted on leadership in a great way. Leaders were dying, and so were the people in the upper class. Consequently, Aurelius, in his letter to Athens in 174 A.D., loosened the qualification for one to enter the Areopagus. This was the Council of Athens. It was a great honor and prestige to belong to this council. The inclusion of other classes other than the upper class ensured more representation of different classes in the council and was a huge political step towards democracy. The plague was considered a punishment from the gods. In an attempt to appease them, the Romans built more temples and other places of worship. The crisis affected the people psychologically. The people were emotionally exhausted from suffering grief and anxiety. Moreover, most of them had lost faith in many things; their army- they were facing attacks from foreigners; religion- they hoped for a cure from the gods, but none of them was quick to provide one; the leadership- leaders were dying as well as the civilians. In short, this was a very tough era for the Romans. They were facing abject poverty because most people could not work, and commodities were too expensive. Poverty impacted the feeling of desperateness in the people's minds. During the Antonine Plague, everyone was living in fear and grief. It was one of the darkest ages in the history of the Roman Empire. During such a crisis, good leadership is key to controlling fear that the people have and calming the citizens down. Stoicism played a significant role in comforting the people and giving them hope. Stoicism is the act of enduring pain and hardship without complaining. It was founded in Athens in the 3rd century AD by Zenus of Citium. By the time the plague struck Rome, there were many Stoics, and Marcus Aurelius was one of them. They reminded the people to remain calm and endure as the plague too would pass.

Marcus Aurelius encouraged his people; he told them that the disease would come to an end. He said, 'Time is a sort of river of passing events, and strong is its current; no sooner is a thing brought to sight than it is swept by and another takes its place, and this too will be swept away.' He urged them to be fearless by saying, 'It is not death that a man should fear, but he should fear never beginning to live.' He encouraged them to keep on striving every day when he uttered, 'the art of living is more like wrestling than dancing.' In the shadow of misfortune, he reminded them to be grateful when he said, 'When you arise in the morning, think of what a precious privilege it is to be alive- to breathe, to think, to enjoy, to love.' Unfortunately, the plague struck the empire, and in 180 A.D., he passed on. He was 58 years old. This was yet another blow to the empire. Commodus, his son, succeeded him as emperor. The Antonine Plague died with Marcus Aurelius. It claimed 20 million lives, which was about 10% of the population of Rome. Rome recovered from this in 279 AD. This plague was one of the turning points in the History of the Roman Empire. It plunged Rome into a period of downfall from which it would never recover. Such is the power of pandemics. They bring about economic, political, and social problems that were never foreseen. For people to understand the gravity of a problem, they have to live through it. As modern citizens of the world, we have come to realize that pandemics will hit the world as long as microorganism species keep on evolving and as new species will attack us. How are we prepared socially, economically, and scientifically in the face of such calamity? Will we crumble? Will we stand strong and respond well to the pandemic? Will we be the first generation in history to find a cure in time and survive? Will we let only the strong survive, or shall we stand united as a species?

Dracunculus Medinensis

The name Dracunculus medinensis roughly translates to 'the fiery dragon of Medina.' Its common name is Guinea worm, and it causes dracunculiasis, dracontiasis or the Guinea Worm Disease. It is uncommon in our world today because the World Health Organization continues to fight to eradicate this disease. In some countries, people are paid when they report it. It is a nematode, a roundworm. The female grows up to 80cm long while the male, which is not so long, grows up to 4cm. The worm was described in Egypt as early as in the 15th Century BC in the Ebers papyrus. In the Bible, it was probably mentioned as the fiery serpents that plagued the Israelites near the Red Sea. In the Ebers papyrus, there is a description of the clinical manifestation of the disease, which included blisters, instructions for treating the swelling, and the removal of worms from arms and legs. Physicians were conversant with the morphology and the effects of the disease. Historians doubt that they knew the connection of the disease with water. It may have been endemic to different places in the past. For instance, there are the 7th-century Assyrian texts that describe dracunculiasis in detail. The texts were found in the ancient city of Nineveh, in the library of King Ashurbanipal. Galen of Pergamum, a physician, and Plutarch, a writer, documented dracontiasis in ancient Greece. The disease resurged in Africa and Asia, and travelers began seeing it in 1674. Scientists studied the life cycle of Dracunculus medinensis but did not quite understand it. In 1870, Aleksei Pavlovich Fedchenko, a Russian scientist, discovered the intermediary crustacean stages, thus making a major break-through as far as understanding the lifecycle of the worm is concerned. In 1913, Dyneshvar Atmaran, an Indian bacteriologist, confirmed the findings of Fedchenko when he successfully infected people with the Guinea Worm Disease using infected water fleas. Parasitologists continued to study the Guinea worm, and they realized that the disease could be easily avoided due to its water-based life. Since the extraction of the worm, it was coiled around a stick, and it is contended that the serpent around the healing staff of Asclepius, the Greco-Roman god of medicine, is a Guinea worm rather than a snake. Despite never having encountered the disease, Galen is credited with the coining of the term dracontiasis. Some scientists and physicians are rumored to have mistaken the Guinea worm for a protruding nerve. This includes Ambroise Pare of France. In the 1970s, a calcified guinea worm was found in a male mummy, which dated back to 1000 BC. This confirmed the existence of Guinea worm disease in the ancient world. The ancient Greeks established the relationship between water and the disease. The worm is most commonly found in subtropical and tropical regions. The temperatures in these areas are mostly about 27 degrees Celsius (27°C), and rarely undergo fluctuation. This provides the perfect condition for the development of the larvae. In the 1980s, Guinea Worm Disease (GWD) was prevalent and endemic in some countries in Africa and Asia. However, today, only a few countries still have cases of this disease. It has been reported in South West Asia like Iran, Iraq, Pakistan, among others. The World Health Organization reported a total of 54 cases in four countries; Angola, Chad, South Sudan, and Cameroun. All of these countries are in Africa. The worm is water-based. Water fleas, also known as copepods, are the primary vectors of this nematode. They are crustaceans. Water fleas are found in salty and fresh water. They feed on the larvae of the guinea worm. After being ingested, the larva develops into the infective stage within two weeks and passing via two molt stages. Humans then consume water infested with the fleas, which are mostly found in water from stagnant places. The gastric juice and hydrochloric acid in the digestive system then digested the copepods, and the larvae are released into the stomach. The males and the females move by boring through the tissues. In the tissues, they grow and attain maturity, and then mate. The males then die immediately after mating. Almost one year after infection, a blister appears on the skin of the victim, and then one or two female worms appear. The worms mainly appear on the legs and feet. This is accompanied by a burning sensation, and that is why this roundworm is referred to as a dragon. While extracting, the part is dipped in water to relieve this sensation. The female worm then releases other ineffective larvae into the water. The larvae are fed on by the copepods, and the cycle continues. Infection occurs mostly during the dry season, in humid climates, or during drought. In the semiarid, wet and dry climates, it occurs just after the rainy season. In both cases, copepods grow rapidly because of the lower water surface of stationary bodies. Symptoms only appear just prior to the worm's emergence. The symptoms include fever and swelling in the part of the body where the worm is located. A blister forms excruciatingly, showing that a worm is just about to emerge. This makes the disease hard to control. It is, therefore, a silent invader and even a more disastrous annihilator. This disease is a menace because even though it is rarely fatal, it has debilitating effects and cripples people for life. It causes problems with the limbs. Moving the limbs even slightly becomes horribly excruciating. This renders some people unproductive, especially if they do manual work or work that requires the person to move about. There are a lot of stigmas associated with Guinea Worm Disease, especially in African communities where it was endemic. It is considered disgusting, and for communities that didn't understand it, it was a sign of impurity and ill intentions. As the worms were being expelled, the person was considered to be undergoing sanctification. Let's take a scenario; there's a man named Joseph, aged 25 years. He is working as a chauffeur and is about to marry his fiancée. He suddenly comes down with Guinea Worm Disease. Eventually, he becomes incapacitated. He gets dismissed from his job as he is no longer able to do it. His fiancée now thinks he is not her type and calls off the wedding. This shows how devastating this disease can be. There is not yet a vaccine or a cure for Dracunculiasis. This means that the only way that people can solve this malady is by prevention. After all, prevention is better than cure. People have to drink safe and clean water. Failure to do this exposes them to the water flea, and consequently, the disease. People have to heighten surveillance such that the first worm detected is reported. But assuming that the worm is first detected as it is being extracted from a person, is it not a bit late because other people may have drunk or could still be drinking the contaminated water? How effective is this as a mode of prevention of this illness? After a worm has already been detected, the transmission of the disease from the worm should be prevented. This should be done by regularly cleaning and bandaging the affected areas of the skin until the worms have been completely expelled from the body. The infected persons should be prevented from wading through the water to avoid contamination of the water by the ineffective larvae. There should be improved access to clean and safe drinking water to avoid the infection of the people. If all the people have to drink water from open water bodies, they have to take necessary measures to ensure that the water is safe for use. They may do this by filtering or boiling. They may also kill the water fleas by spraying the water with chemicals. To kill the larvae of the water fleas, they should use larvicides. Knowledge is the strongest weapon in the fight against dracontiasis. It promotes behavioral change and protects the people. The World Health Organization has almost successfully eradicated Guinea Worm Disease. This has taken cooperation between the organization, state, health workers, and the affected communities. The first and most important step is the education of the community concerning the pathology and the life cycle of this disease. They help them understand that the most effective way of curbing the disease is by either killing the larvae or the primary vector, the copepods. The journey to elimination started in 1981 when the Interagency Steering Committee for the International Drinking Water Supply and Sanitation Decade proposed elimination of

Guinea Worm Disease as an indication of the success of the decade. This was to happen between 1981 and 1990. The World Health Assembly adopted this resolution and acted with the Interagency Steering Committee for the International Drinking Water Supply. Other bodies such as the United States Centers for Disease Control and Prevention and The Carter Center joined the battle against this disease. The WHO and United States Centers for Disease Control and Prevention formulated technical guidelines on how to eradicate this disease. This included facts about the disease and measures of its prevention. WHO coordinates eradication activities and also enforces surveillance. Between 1980 and 2011, only 20 countries have been endemic to Dracunculiasis. WHO is the only organization that can certify that a country is free to this disease following recommendations by the ICCDE. ICCDE is an international body of public health officers. For a country to be declared free of Guinea Worm Disease, it has to have zero cases of transmission and maintain active surveillance of the disease for at least 3 consecutive years. The duration ensures that no cases have been missed, and this prevents the re-occurrence of the disease. If a single case is missed, it may delay eradication of the disease by a year or more, since the incubation period is 12-14 months. Pieces of evidence of the re-emergence of this disease have been reported in Ethiopia (2008) after the national eradication program had already claimed that they had interrupted the transmission of the disease. In Chad, the disease re-occurred after the country had reported zero cases for 10 years. This was demoralizing. A country that reports zero cases for 14 months enters the precertification phase. It is said to have interrupted the transmission of the disease. The country remains in this phase for 3 consecutive years since the last indigenous case reported. During this period, intensive surveillance is carried out. Even after the country is declared free of Guinea Worm Disease, continuous and intensive surveillance has to continue to detect and avoid reoccurrence until global eradication is declared. There have been challenges that have been encountered in the journey of eradication. As the fight against the disease was starting, the idea was that the disease was only in humans. However, the disease was also detected in carnivores. Some animals, such as dogs, have been detected with Guinea worms. These worms are genetically identical to those that emerge from human beings. This phenomenon was reported in Chad in 2012. Other countries experiencing this problem are Ethiopia and Mali. The dogs posed a challenge in the eradication of the disease since the animals are hard to control and survey, especially when the disease has not already been detected in them. To understand the magnitude of this problem, we have to understand that in 2019 Chad reported 1,935 infected dogs and 46 infected cats. Ethiopia had 2 infected dogs and six infected baboons. Mali reported 9 infected dogs. Angola had one infected dog. WHO has given some guidelines on how to deal with the challenge of canine infections. There should be enhanced surveillance to detect all infected animals and contain them successfully. To effectively contain the animals, there should be tethering of the infected animals and proactive tethering. Proactive tethering involves animals that may have consumed water from the contaminated source or animals in the entire endangered area. The most expensive and challenging step in the eradication of the disease is finding and containing the last cases. This is because the disease occurs in very remote areas that are not only difficult to access but also full of insecurity. There has been a remarkable success in the journey to the eradication of the Guinea Worm Disease. This is because of cooperation between the community members, the health sectors of the affected countries, and the World Health Organization. This shows that when everybody plays their part, even the greatest burden becomes just a feather. Education that is offered to the community members ensures that they are at the forefront of curbing the disease. The measures could be taken as a model during the fight for the eradication of other diseases, especially water-based and water-borne diseases. If we can eradicate this disease, so can we eliminate others that continue to scourge the earth.

The Plague of Athens

Epidemic and pandemic are Greek words in origin. This tells us that the Greeks must have experienced outbreaks of pestilences. During the Peloponnesian War, the Athenians were at war against the Spartans in an attempt to establish dominance over them. In the second year of this war (430 BC), there was an outbreak of a disease that would persist until when it would die out four years later. This plague is considered the most lethal in the classical Greek History. For a city that was already in crisis, the disease had an unfortunate timing. It put the Athenians to the test and exposed the cracks and fractures that were in their way of life. Their morals, their religion, their government, basically, the whole society. The epidemic started in Sub-Saharan Africa, south of Ethiopia. It then spread northwards and westwards. It became a pandemic that hit Egypt and swept through Libya. It also swept across the Mediterranean Sea into Persia and eventually to Greece, where it would shatter the city of Athens. The Plague entered the city of Athens via the Port of Piraeus. It is one of the most remembered plagues that ever hit this city. Thucydides recorded this pestilence in detail in his book, 'The History of the Peloponnesian war (431-404 BC).' He not only lived through the pandemic but also suffered from it and survived. Thucydides, the father of political realism, assessed the plague in all its dimensions. How it affected the society socially, economically, and politically. Despite his lack of knowledge in medicine, Thucydides vividly documented the symptoms of the plague. This was to ensure that if this disease strikes again, the people would recognize it and find remedies or a cure to it. The patients had a fever. This sounds normal because our bodies raise temperatures to kill the invading microbes. However, the fever that Thucydides describe was so high that the patients asked to be stark naked. Even the lightest piece of linen was uncomfortable for them. Some preferred to be submerged in cold water to relieve the heat. The body was not hot when touched, despite the inferno that was raging in the inside. The patients did not appear pale but reddish and livid. The patients also had an insatiable thirst that could not be quenched by any amounts of water or any other liquids. The thirst could have resulted from the profuse sweating of the patients. He describes the patients as being tormented by an unceasing thirst that was utterly insatiable. The throat, tongue, and other internal organs of the patients were inflamed. Moreover, they produced an unnatural, fetid breath. The patient then started sneezing and had hoarseness. They would cough and feel so much pain in the chest. The patients were restless and had insomnia. The patients would have muscle spasms, which most people thought was the bodies' struggle against the internal inflammation. The patients also suffered from terrible backaches, and violent abdominal pain; there were digestive juices that were secreted during this ailment. Most patients would die a painful death after 7-9 days from the onset of the symptoms. The illness, however, left the body's strength intact. If the patients were fortunate enough to survive the first phase of this disease, they would have violent ulceration. Thucydides observed that numerous pustules would emerge from the livid body of the patient, thereby causing severe diarrhea, which usually resulted in their death. This could probably be due to dehydration that may have resulted from diarrhea and loss of water from the skin, which was damaged by the pustules. Those who survived the disease suffered from a great deal of disfigurement. Their genitals, fingers, and toes were defaced, at times lost. The victims lost sight, and some became deaf and dumb. The effect that clobbered most patients was the loss of memory. Thucydides describes that they lost knowledge of their friends, and sadly, of themselves. The sickness plagued every part of the body, and it devoured the patients' dignity to the bones. Birds and other animals that normally fed on the corpses would be repelled by those of the victims of this pestilence. Those that preyed on these corpses would either disappear or be found dead. Some would die from just tasting the corpse.

Therefore, everyone, man, and some beasts avoided coming into contact with the bodies, even though so many were left unburied. Thucydides says that the streets were filled with corpses lying upon each other, and half-dead creatures could be seen crawling towards fountains with a great longing for water. The virulence of this disease and the viciousness of the symptoms showed that it had not been experienced in the past. The number of lives that it also claimed showed that the people had not been exposed to it before the time of the plague. Long ago, the old men of Athens had said, 'A Dorian war shall come and with it, death.' The Athenians felt that these words were being fulfilled during the plague. They were at war with Spartans and were also bearing the weight of a cruel plague that did not care for class or age. One to two hundred thousand people perished due to this disease. This was a large number for a city. This constituted a third of the population. Whole families died as a result of the plague. The people who died were too many, and some of their bodies littered the streets. The people who were already devastated by the death of their soldiers in the Peloponnesian war were downcast. Thanatos, the god of death, was looming in the city and was cutting locks of the people en masse, and with no mercy. Most leaders perished during this pestilence. Athens lost Pericles, who perished along with his wife and two sons. He was a statesman who was responsible for the development and maturation of Athenian democracy and the democracy of the empire. This shook the people and left them with no one to look up to, their ember of equality and justice. He departed when the city needed him most, in the middle of two monster crises. The disease caused the people to die in misery and utter agony. Consequently, people started panicking because the disease spread too fast. Those who were not already infected were anticipating catching the illness. Physicians fell sick due to their frequent and close contact with the ailing and died, and this caused terror to prevail in the people's hearts. Those that got infected became disillusioned and were in utter despair. They lost the resilience to fight the disease due to the hopelessness that was deeply engraved in their hearts. For this reason, many succumbed to the illness. Despair and fear were reigning supreme in these dark days as people fled from the cities to the countryside. The number of people who were arriving in the countryside overwhelmed those that were there. The houses could no longer hold any more people. The people had to lodge in cabins, which were unsanitary and congested. This greatly increased the rate of the spread of disease, and consequently, the death of the people. As the disease continued to devour the 'haves and the have nots,' the chaos started to be experienced in different parts of the city. As the rich people died, ravenous people started taking over their property and using it as their own. They took over their homes, everything in it, and claimed it as theirs. They wanted to use this wealth and enjoy before death claimed them too. This wreaked havoc and lawlessness because many of these people wanted to have a share of the wealth of the people who were dying. The laws concerning honoring of the dead were rarely followed. The coin ceased to be placed in the mouths of the departed. Their bodies were no longer buried or cremated. They were left in the streets for the birds of prey and beasts to devour. All the laws of man or the gods were not followed. The people felt that despite Pericles' attempt to protect the people from the Spartans, they were still perishing within the walls of the city due to the plague. The plague was sparing none, upright or immoral. It was a time of utter anarchy. They were experiencing death within the walls and destruction without. This caused disorder, those who seemed to be people of honor lost their morals. The people who once upheld compassion, now neglected the sick to die. Those who were once kind fled their friends in a quest to save their own lives. The people became selfish. They no longer feared punishment as a result of breaking the law. They said that the disease would agonize them to death even before the gods could strike. People did whatever the law forbade them to do. They stole, plundered, killed, and destroyed. It was a period of distress. People's lives were on the scales. If the plagues didn't take it, the Spartans would. If the Spartans were late to do it, the anarchic citizens would do it. The turbulence that was witnessed during that period was greater than ever before. As Michelle Obama once said, a crisis does not create a new character but only reveals the heathen that is buried deep within people. Thucydides says that those who behaved this way were not moral in the first place. They did what they did in the pretext of being good to avoid the wrath of the gods. Whatever evil men had been doing in dark corners, they now did it in the open. The law enforcement included policemen and was still young. It had also suffered the loss of many members, and those who remained were striving for self-preservation, so there was no restriction to do anything. Many people were suffering from the disease as well as solitude. Their close relations had not only abandoned them but also fled the city. The majority had no one to look after them, and they died. A group of people had their lucky stars shine upon them and survived the monstrosity. They understood what the ailing were going through. They, too, had experienced it, and as they say, experience is the best teacher. They took care of the sick with the utmost care and gave them a ray of hope amidst the growing insanity. Those who survived never caught the disease again, and if they did, it didn't affect them as much as it did during the first attack. Some people chose to take care of the others; they risked their health and life. They felt that it was the right thing to do despite being surrounded by egoists and law-breakers. The Athenians continued to break the law. The plague continued to devour and daze all, upright and immoral, noble and slave, just or corrupt. Everyone was pulling its yoke, and the burden was heavy to bear. These made the people lack faith in their gods. They questioned their intentions if at all, the plague was from them. Some questioned their power, as they could not protect the believers from it. This society was feeling very vulnerable because they were in the middle of a battle with a visible enemy when another unseen enemy attacked. When the plague at Athens died out in 426 BC, it had reaped so many lives, diminished the faith of the majority of the people in their gods, and turned so many people into barbarians who could no longer follow the rule of law. Never before had such lawlessness been witnessed in Athens or Greece as a nation. Therefore, stricter rules were put in place in both religion and the city. Policemen became sterner, laws were more strict and rulers more austere. This was all done to try and bring back the calm, which was the normal state of affairs before the plague struck. Historians and scientists have been trying to identify the mysterious plague that struck Athens. For the last 2500 years, they have been giving suggestions, but up to date, no disease has been pinpointed as the cause of the plague that devoured the ancient city. Some people thought it might have been bubonic plague, but no buboes were mentioned, and this rules it out. Some have said that it was Ergot poisoning as its symptoms were fever, abdominal cramps, diarrhea, all of which were documented by Thucydides. Some suggested smallpox, epidemic typhus, while others suggest that it may have been multiple illnesses. All in all, Thucydides documented the disease so that if it happened in the future, it could be recognized. There is no doubt that it could be recognized, but will we be able to find a cure for it or a vaccine? The plague of Athens and the events that happened makes one wonder, will we as human beings panic in times of crisis as the Athenians did? Will we become reckless and egoists or hold on to our humanity? Will we follow the measures put in place to maintain harmony or crush them beneath our feet? Will we learn from our predecessors' mistakes or wait to learn from our own? Lest we forget that these mistakes cost us lives.

The smallpox epidemic in Japan

Smallpox is said to have originated from India or Egypt at least 3000 years ago. The mummy of Ramses, the pharaoh, was found to be having bumps or pocks on the face, which could have been smallpox. Japan was endemic to smallpox for centuries. They have suffered several outbreaks in the past. The most lethal of all of the outbreaks was the first one, which commenced in 735 A.D. and persisted for 2 years. They called it the epidemic of Tenpyo. Japan had been experiencing outbreaks of infectious diseases due to their increased contact and interaction with the mainland. A few decades before this smallpox epidemic, the government adopted this, and so when the epidemic happened, most people were aware of it. The epidemic started in the city of Dazaifu, Fukuoka, in Northern Kyushu. The infection was carried by Japanese fishermen who had been stranded in the Korean Peninsula. The epidemic spread throughout Northern Kyushu throughout the year and the next. The people died in huge numbers, like flies. Devastated, most people fled the farms in fear of contracting the killer disease. In 736 A.D., the government sent a group of emissaries to Korea. They were to pass through Kyushu. Most of the people in the group contracted the illness and died. This alarmed the survivors in the group, and they went back to the capital at Nara and told the rulers about the horrible disease which had caused deaths of the Northerners and their colleagues. Unknowingly, these officials had spread smallpox to Nara and Eastern Japan. The disease initially caused flu-like symptoms which did not alarm many people. This included high fever, headaches, body aches, and sometimes vomiting. During this period, the people could carry out their normal activities. Very few of the infected people were bed-ridden. An early rash would occur on the fourth day after the onset of the symptoms. It started as small red spots in the mouth and tongue. The spots would then change into sores that would break, spreading large amounts of the virus in the mouth and throat. The person would continue having a fever. A rash would then appear on the skin, starting on the face. It would then spread to the arms and legs. Within a day, the whole body would have the rashes. The rashes became pustules, raised, and filled with thick opaque pus. The pustules would grow to the size of a pea. After some days, the pustules would scab over. The scabs would fall over, leaving marks and pits. They left the person spotted. The scabs would fall off approximately 3 weeks after the rash appeared. Smallpox was fatal to the people in Japan. The viciousness with which it attacked and the sky-high death toll indicates that this was the first time the people had ever encountered it. Smallpox devastated the people of Japan. They believed that it was caused by a mythical creature known as Onryo. This spirit was able to take physical form to seek vengeance among the living. In an attempt to cure this disease, the people tried to scare off the demon. Onryo was believed to be afraid of the color red as well as dogs. The people developed a custom whereby they displayed red dolls, wore red clothing, or painted red during rituals. The people in Okinawa tried to appease this demon. They played the Sanshin, a musical instrument, and performed the lion dance while dressed in a red outfit. They presented flowers and burnt incense to appease the demon. This red treatment became popular, and the physicians insisted that it relieved the symptoms of the illness. It was used in other places far and side. The red treatment was practiced in Europe by Queen Elizabeth when she was wrapped in a red blanket when she suffered an episode of the disease in 1562. As smallpox spread to other parts of the world, so did the red treatment, Erythro Therapy. Niels Finsen, a Nobel laureate, gave it scientific authority. He claimed the red light reduced the severity of the scarring. People held this to be true until researchers proved it wrong. In China, the gods of smallpox had to be appeased to avoid catching the illness. In West Africa, the smallpox god, Sopona, who was associated with red, was also honored to avoid the disease. The Christians in Europe were advised to lead a pious life to avoid this sickness. Some people were fortunate enough to survive this epidemic. They got well despite the viciousness with which the disease attacked. It was observed that they never suffered the disease again. They survived to tell the tale of the misery they went through because of the pestilence. They were therefore urged to nurse victims of the pestilence back to health, for it was known that no one could contact the disease twice. The epidemic had so much impact in this community that had never experienced it before. In a quest to avoid the vengeance of Onryo, the people fled their farms and homes. At the end of 736 AD, Kyushu was already experiencing great famine. The lack of a proper diet meant that the people's immunity was dwindling, and this made the blow of the disease even harder for them to bear. As some people died and others fled, agriculture failed terribly in virtually all parts of Japan. There was an imbalance of labor because some places were densely populated, and others were sparsely populated. This meant that some places had no one to cultivate crops, while others had too many people. The impact was so hard that at the end of the epidemic, the government leased land to private owners who were willing to cultivate. They did this in an attempt to improve agriculture and, consequently, the economy. This partly reinvigorated the communities to work and try to regain the empire's lost glory. The epidemic struck far and wide, affecting all levels of society. Leaders, also known as court nobles, suffered from smallpox and died due to it. For instance, the powerful Fujiwara clan lost all of the four brothers to the pandemic. This denied them political leverage as they were overtaken by their longtime rival Tachibana no Moroe. It wreaked havoc among all, princes or paupers. It took at least one-third of the population as it affected all segments of the population; the young children, youth, the middle-aged, and the adults. This was very unfortunate, considering that the empire's economy depended on farming and construction. This was not helped by the fact that most survivors were weak and bed-ridden, the majority of them breathing their last. The epidemic took away at least one-third of Japan's population. This included all young and old. As the disease was being blamed upon the demon Onryo, the people felt that their refuge and salvation would be in Buddha. The emperor Shomu felt a personal responsibility for the smallpox pandemic. He embarked on building temples and statues for the god. The grand temple was constructed at Todai-Ji. He also built other temples in other provinces. Many people, therefore, started practicing Buddhism, and up to date, Japan is home to a huge population of indigenous Buddhists. The epidemic weakened the people, decimating their capacity to work and pay taxes. At the peak of the epidemic, emperor Shomu declared a tax waiver for everyone during this period of great distress. Some of the regions were totally exempted from paying taxes at all. It took a great deal of time and effort for the country to have a steady economy. The epidemic was just but a beginning of outbreaks of the disease but none as lethal as the first. This is partial because those who survived had developed acquired immunity. By the 1200s, Japan had already experienced 28 outbreaks of this disease. The Japanese villages were struck by the pestilence every ten years. Therefore, they sought measures to prevent the disease or to mollify its symptoms. As expected, the disease did not affect all the parts of this vast land in the same way, and different communities had different ways of dealing with the disease. Villages in the central area of the empire were hit more times by this epidemic. They made sacrifices to the smallpox demons regularly to avoid their wrath. They also made it a habit to decorate their homes in red and to wear red clothing. However, the malady still struck despite all these measures. When it did, it was the responsibility of everyone to use magical and religious methods that they knew to treat the sick. The peripheral regions were rarely affected by this disease. Unfortunately, when it did, it attacked with maliciousness, took so many lives, and weakened the individuals in a way that astonished the people from the central regions. The villagers of the peripheral regions responded to the malady by spatial quarantine, which was basically fleeing from the patients. This proved effective to them as it protected a segment of their healthy but vulnerable population. This astonished the people from the central region. They saw it as immoral and barbaric. As the years went by, the outbreaks started affecting the infants and young children, and it caused their deaths. This was because the majority of adults had already been infected with the disease and developed immunity against it. The majority of the children died because maybe at the time of the outbreak, their immunity was not yet well-developed to fight it off. Getting the pox became a rite of passage. After contracting it and getting well, there would be a celebration for they had escaped death. In an attempt to infect their children, some parents would have planned what would be a pox party today. As smallpox continued to wreak terror in different places of the globe, more effective measures were put in place by different communities in an attempt to cure or to get ready before the virus could get to them. In Asia, medics came up with variolation. This was whereby one would be deliberately infected with the disease. Sounds familiar? Dried smallpox scabs would be blown into the nose of an individual. This way, they would contract a mild form of the illness, and upon recovery, they would be immune to the disease. Some people died in the process but most recovered. The death toll was only 3%, which was mild compared to 30% of people who died if they contracted the malady naturally. By 1700, variolation was practiced in Africa, India, and the Ottoman Empire. Unlike in Africa and Asia, in Europe, the dried scabs were placed under the skin rather than being blown into the nose. This method became popular, and many people were protected from the virus. In 1796, Edward Jenner developed the first vaccine against smallpox. It was the first vaccine to have ever been created. He took the pus from the pustules of a milk-maid who was suffering from cow-pox. He weakened it and injected his gardener's son. After several days, he exposed him to smallpox deliberately, but he did not get sick. At first, everyone thought his idea was wild, but when he tried it on his wife, and she never got sick, people started slowly but surely using it. Today vaccination is one of the surest ways to evade a disease. Smallpox continued to inflict different communities in the world. It caused terror and huge losses. The World Health Organization declared war against smallpox. They aimed to eradicate the illness. Mass vaccination programs were the main weapons against this monstrosity. As they say, prevention is better than cure; they were aware that if people were vaccinated, they would not have to experience the agony that this disease caused. The last known person to have the disease was Ali Maow Maalin, from Somalia. In the 33rd General Assembly of WHO, on May 8, 1980, the world was declared free of Smallpox. Smallpox caused terror in Japan and changed their lives socially, economically, and religiously. Only a few places have been allowed to store the smallpox virus for research purposes. World Health Organization conducts awareness programs of what to do if the virus reemerges. People have fear that it could be used as a biological weapon. Will it wreak terror as it did in Japan and take a multitude of lives? Will it change people's lifestyles? How will the world of better technology and vast medical knowledge react to it? Have the people forgotten all about it, or are they ready for the re-emergence of an enemy that once scourged their predecessors?

Spanish Flu

The deadliest influenza pandemic in recent history occurred in 1918. You may not have heard about it as it was overshadowed by the First World War, which was at its peak. It was caused by the influenza virus of subtype H1N1 origin. It is speculated that the virus was of avian origin. It is not clear where the disease originated but despite its name, it did not originate from Spain. Spain, which was a neutral country during the ongoing World War, was the first to admit that there was a strange malady in its territory. Three theories postulated where the flu might have originated. The first theory says that the disease may have started in a military camp at Camp Funston in Kansas. This is because, in March 1918, a cook, Albert Gitchell, who worked in this camp, was hospitalized after being confirmed to have the illness; many soldiers got infected. The soldiers from America spread the deadly virus to Europe when they fought in the World War on the Western Front. The second theory speculates that the disease started in Southern China, in Guangdong Province. The disease affected laborers, who then spread it to America and Europe. In Europe, they were digging trenches during the war. The third theory hypothesizes that this flu started with the soldiers on the Western Front between 1916 and 1917, independent of any diffusion from China or America. The soldiers lived in what would be considered the accurate description of an unhealthy living space; damp, congested, and unsanitary. The disease, therefore, spread quickly throughout the ranks, and some recovered after 3 days, but unfortunately, some died. At the end of the World War, the soldiers carried the flu home and obviously spread it very quickly. The Spanish flu pandemic attacked the world in three waves. The first wave started in March 1918 and was mild compared with the other waves. The flu affected people, young and old, indiscriminately. The flu or influenza is a virus that attacks the respiratory tract. The first wave of the disease is characterized by symptoms of the typical flu. This includes fever, chills, and fatigue. The mortality rate was low, and so the disease was not an issue in the shadow of the World War. The second wave of the pandemic occurred in the fall of 1918. It was far more lethal than the first wave. It was a mutated influenza virus. The scientists who studied the genome of the virus found out that the disease had more capacity to attack and disrupt the upper respiratory tract making way for bacterial pneumonia. The patients who would complain of flu symptoms would be dead within 24 hours at the most. The new strain was highly contagious and was spread through air droplets released when an infected person was coughing, sneezing, or talking. The virus could survive outside the human body, on surfaces. People who touch these surfaces and then touch their mouths, noses, and eyes contract it. The disease caused fever, chills, and difficulty in breathing. Unlike the other waves of this flu, the second wave was more lethal to the young people at the prime of their lives (20-40 years old) rather than the very young or the very old. For instance, in the USA, soldiers would be admitted in large numbers, and in the morning, their dead bodies would be lying like cold wood in the morgue. In America, the life expectancy in 1917 was 51 years but had dropped to 39 years in 1918 due to the rate at which the young people were perishing. Scientists learned that this was due to a phenomenon known as cytokine explosion. This is the overreaction of the immune system against the influenza virus. The stronger the immune system, the higher the rate of the cytokine explosion, and that explains why the second wave mainly affected the young people. Cytokine explosion was characterized by the filling of fluid in the lungs. The people drowned in this fluid, and their strong immune systems were now acting against them. The second wave of influenza was characterized by the skin turning blue due to hypoxia. This is the lack of oxygen in the tissues due to the malfunctioning of the lungs. There were other pneumonia-related complications, such as bronchitis and ear and sinus infections. This type of pneumonia was referred to as atypical pneumonias. Today we call them Acute

Respiratory Distress Syndrome (ARDS). The second wave of the Spanish flu spread with the speed of lightning. It occurred at the peak of the war during which troops of soldiers were moving en masse from one area to the other. The soldiers had poor living conditions. There was a shortage of food in the military camps, and this had affected their immunity, decimating it. They were living in damp, congested places, which were dirty and did not have enough water. This increased the rate at which the disease spread. Some civilians were living in such conditions, whether in refugee camps or their own homes, and this did not help the situation. Some communities experienced the lethargy of this monstrosity in its rawest form. For instance, the village of Brevig Mission in Alaska, had a population of about 100 people. The town lost 90% of its population. Philadelphia, Pennsylvania, USA, was also struck hard by the pandemic. The flu arrived in the Philadelphia Navy Yard in September 1918 when 600 sailors arrived from Boston. They then became sick 4 days later. By October 1, there were 635 new cases, and within no time, it was the city with the highest death toll in the USA. It has been speculated that the city did not take precautions; in a nutshell, they did not effect a lock-down. About 16,000 people died in the city, and about 675,000 Americans died overall. The city, like the rest of America, was experiencing a shortage of medical personnel because most of them were in Europe taking care of the soldiers in the ongoing World War. The second wave contributed the most number of deaths during the pandemic. Influenza affected human beings, poultry, and swine. Several factors contributed to the rapid spread of the second wave of the disease; the main reason was that there was no quarantine as there was an on-going war. In some places such as Britain, the leaders knew that a lockdown was necessary due to the looming danger of the pestilence. Nevertheless, they did not implement it, for the war had to be fought. The tools that were used to study microbiology, such as microscopes, could not view viruses. The people did not understand what viruses were, their structure, or how they propagated. The people had neither vaccines nor antiviral therapies to combat the illness. The first licensed vaccine against influenza was made in 1940. The medical personnel thought that the disease was caused by bacteria. The antibiotics that could probably treat the bacteria were 10 years from being discovered. The hospitals were overwhelmed by the increasing number of patients. With the scarcity of medical personnel, the patients were overcrowded, and this only worsened the situation. The medical personnel caught the flu, and the situation was helpless. In that era, the media was mainly focusing on the war, where the governments channeled most of their resources. In some parts of the world, people were not aware of the magnitude of the disease they were dealing with. This caused the rapid spread of the disease to the people who were unaware of this dire situation. The Spanish media was impartial in the dissemination of the news, and this played a critical role in the awareness of the pandemic. Most countries in Europe and the world were under censorship regimes, and this limited the spread of life-saving information about the flu pandemic. The people, therefore, tried non-pharmaceutical solutions to control the illness. Some places implemented quarantines and lockdowns. In some parts of America, some scouts arrested those who violated the quarantine and accused them of breaking the Sanitary Code. For instance, St Louis, Missouri closed schools, movie theaters, and public gatherings and only experienced about 2000 deaths. Citizens in places such as San Francisco were allowed to go in public but only when wearing masks. Failure to do so would lead to a fine of $5, which was a significant amount back then. Doctors were at a loss on how to combat the pestilence. They started recommending remedies that they thought would relieve the symptoms. They had been used to combat normal flu in the past. The remedies included beef broth, chicken soup, cinnamon, and drinking wine. Mints were recommended for young children; they were to suck 5 tablets per day to inhibit the infectious process. They also recommended aspirin, which has been blamed for the number of deaths that sky-rocketed in October. The American doctors asked people to stay indoors to avoid shaking hands and to avoid touching the face and eyes. Furthermore, they asked the libraries to stop lending books and for people to wear masks. The second wave wreaked havoc in the four corners of the globe. It was in Europe, America, Asia, and Africa. About 1.8-1.9 billion people were infected. The death toll was so high that the morgues were overwhelmed. The cemeteries were filled up, and eventually, the people had to bury their deceased family members themselves. In some places such as Brevig Mission, they had to bury their people in mass graves. There were 50-100 million deaths worldwide. This was about a third of the world's population. This means that the plague was more of a menace than the Black Death and the Cyprian plague. The only plague that could match its viciousness was the Justinian plague. This meant that the workforce reduced and essential services such as garbage collection, health services, farm workers, and summer harvest could not be effectively done. The third wave of the disease occurred in the winter and spring of 1919. The virus was less virulent than that of the second wave. The people who had recovered from the previous bout developed immunity to this strain. Those who were affected were the older people who were above 65 years of age and the very young whose immunity was not yet developed. After the discovery of viruses, many scientists were intrigued, particularly Johan Hultin. He was a student at university when he first went to Brevig Mission, excavated a mass grave, and studied the lungs of those who had died due to the Spanish Flu, but he did not establish the cause of the disease then. He re-embarked on the research in 1997 and successfully proved that the disease was viral. This pandemic has been compared to the 2020 Coronavirus pandemic. In terms of the method of spread, they are the same. They have the same effect of causing respiratory distress. The advantage of this pandemic is that the microbe is well understood and can, therefore, be effectively combated. Due to the well-developed machines and techniques, the structure of the virus has been well understood. The pandemic can be well contained if the effective measures are to be taken. The fate is in our hands, literally and figuratively.

Tuberculosis

Tuberculosis is probably the first disease ever to afflict humanity. It is also known as Phthisis, the Consumption, or the White Plague. The causative agent, Mycobacterium tuberculosis, has been detected in remains that date back 9,000 years. That was before any form of human civilization had taken place. It first infected human beings in Africa. Human beings spread it to domestic animals such as cows and goats. The disease then spread along trade routes to other continents, mainly Asia and Europe. Sea lions and seals along the African beaches are believed to have contracted the disease from either humans or animals. They swam across the Atlantic Ocean and transmitted the bacterium to pre-Columbus America. The strain that affects the majority of the Americans has also been found in seals' fossils. By that time, the disease had gained hold of the four corners of the globe, and it was just a matter of wreaking terror and destroying lives. The condition, other than causing the death of many, influenced cultures and religion. Evidence for tuberculosis infection was found in the fossils of human beings who belonged to the Neolithic period. The Neolithic bones showed angulation of bones, which is characteristic of tuberculosis. Molecular methods were used by the scientists to establish the presence of Mycobacterium tuberculosis. In Egypt, signs of this disease have been found in mummies, which date between 3000-2400 BC. The mummy of priest Nesperehen had psoas abscess, which is a sure sign of one having the illness. The mummy of another priest, Philoc, along with other mummies found in the cemetery of Thebes, could have also suffered from tuberculosis. Pharaoh Akhenaten and his wife Nefertiti seem to have died of this ailment. The Eber Papyrus, which dates back to 1500 BC, documents a pulmonary consumption. One characteristic of the disease is that it causes swelling of the cervical lymph nodes. The physicians should perform surgical lancing of the cyst and apply a ground mixture. The mixture consists of seyal, acacia, peas, fruit, honey, salt, animal blood, and insect blood. The disease was very dreaded. In the Old Testament, it is one of the curses that the people would experience if they strayed away from God. Tuberculosis has afflicted each part of the world at different times. In Ancient India, it plagued the people. They referred to the disease as yaksma or Balasa. They were the first to document scrofula, around 1500 BC. Scrofula is also known as Mycobacterial cervical lymphadenitis. This refers to the inflammation of the lymph nodes found in the neck region. The Sushruta Samhita, a document written around 600 BC, recommends the following to be used to treat yaksma; breast milk, alcohol, various meats, among others. The Chinese were also affected by the disease. They described it as Pulmonary Consumption characterized by a weak persistent cough that led to the release of phlegm, fever, a faint but fast pulse, chest obstructions, and shortness of breath. The patients of this sickness were said to have an abnormal appearance. The Chinese believed that the disease caused the person to be empty and void with illness. They also said that the person would reach an incurable state in which the person just waited for death to take over. They are said to be the first people to find out retrospectively, that the disease caused Consumption or damage to the lungs. The Zhou Hou Bei Ji Fang or the Handbook of Prescriptions for Emergencies is one of the earliest documents to mention the symptoms and contagion of tuberculosis. The disease had from 36-99 different kinds of symptoms. The common symptoms were high fever, sweating, asthenia, and pain throughout the body. The condition would linger in the person's lifetime until it would cause their death. It was observed that the disease would also inflict the family members and other people in that household and would finally wipe them out. To cure the disease, the Chinese would use thirty-six charms. The physicians would burn the charms and instruct the patient to inhale the fumes. The fumes had a pungent, unpleasant smell that was not pleasing to the patient, but they had to inhale it nonetheless. The patient would cough out phlegm or vomit until the lousy humor was off the body. However, when the wicked element was out, it was not necessary to continue with fumigation. If the patient happened to die, it was essential to submit all of their belongings to the priest. The priest would burn the belongings together with charms as camouflage to ensure that no one else would use these items, thus reducing the number of new cases. Hippocrates also witnessed this disease in classical times. He and other physicians believed that phthisis was hereditary. In his book, Of the Epidemics, he documented the symptoms of the illness. They include; fever, colorless urine, cough resulting in thick sputa, and loss of appetite and thirst. The loss of appetite resulted in wasting of the muscles and general weakness. Aristotle thought that the disease was contagious. Galen studied the disease and proposed treatments which included; opium as a pain-reliever and as a sleeping agent, blood-letting, and a diet of barley water, fruits, and fish. He described phyma as a tumor in the lung. This could be interpreted as the tubercles which are caused by tuberculosis. Aretaeus vigorously described the symptoms of this disease. He said that the disease caused the voice to be hoarse, the neck slightly bent, tender but not flexible. The fingers became slender because of the wasting of the flesh. However, the joints remained enlarged. The nails of the finger became crooked, and their pulp was shriveled and flat. The nose became sharp and slender; the cheeks became prominent and red. The eyes were hollow, brilliant, and glittering. In the Middle Ages, there was little progress that was made concerning the illness. The physicians continued to believe that the disease was contagious and extremely difficult to treat. Arnaldus de la Villa Nova described the disease as caused by dripping of cold humor from the head to the lungs. In Hungary, the pagans believed that the disease was caused by possession by a dog-shaped demon that attacked the lungs. The people continued to suffer and die from this disease as the physicians struggled to understand this disease and to cure it. The Christians believed that their leaders had divine magic.

They could touch and heal those with the White Plague. It was called the Royal touch and was very popular in France and England. The first touching ceremony was very informal. King Henry IV of France used to perform it once a week after Holy Communion. The spread of the disease in France and England necessitated that the leaders plan more time for the Royal touch. It was propagandized that those who got the Royal touch got healed. This ritual went for a long time, and by 1633, the Book of Common Prayer of the Anglican church had a section for the Royal touch ceremony. One cannot help but wonder, of what medicinal value was the Royal touch? Why did the scientists continue tolerating it if they knew that it added no value to the patients' lives? In this period, Girolamo Fracastoro wrote a book known as De Contagion. In this book, he suggested that tuberculosis was caused by an invisible virus. The virus wrecked the insides of a person. He further noted that it could be spread from one person to the next via direct contact or forms. He also documented that the virus was found on the things that the patient used, such as clothing. It could survive on these clothes for two or three years. However, they did not understand how the disease could propagate for long distances. Paracelsus had a different theory, which he called the Tartaric process. He proposed that every organ had an alchemical duty. The state of complete health could only be attained if each organ fulfilled its duty. If the lungs failed to do so, this would lead to the formation of stone precipitates in the lungs leading to tuberculosis. Major steps were taken in understanding tuberculosis in the 17th and 18th centuries. Franciscus Sylvius realized that; skin ulcers resembled the tubercles seen in the lungs when one was suffering from phthisis. He, therefore, differentiated pulmonary and ganglion tuberculosis. Another scientist Richard Morton proposed that the Consumption was caused by sugar or acidity in the blood. The disease became common in that anyone who got old without contracting the disease became a subject of admiration. Benjamin Marten suggested that the cause of tuberculosis was small microscopic organisms known as animalcules. This was in agreement with the discovery of Anton van Leeuwenhoek, who had observed microscopic organisms. Marten proposed that the animalcules could live in the human body and cause the disease. The people rejected this and continued to shun it for 162 years when Robert Koch finally approved and proved this theory. In 1762, tuberculosis meningitis was explained by Robert Whytt. Percivall Pott described tuberculosis spondylitis, which caused lesions of the vertebrae. It bears his name today. It was in this period that percussion was used as a method of diagnosing the White Plague. This method was also used to tell the extent to which the lungs were damaged. The incidences of tuberculosis accumulated day by day in the Middle Ages. Eventually, it displaced leprosy as the disease that affected. The people were living in small congested places and were migrating to places that were becoming industrialized. This created the perfect environment at which healthy people would contract the illness. Places that were initially free of the disease were now being affected. Whole families and villages were wiped out by the Consumption. It continued to be a disease that puzzled and flustered mankind. A disease causes stigma and shame, but this was not the case with tuberculosis in the 19th century. Those who contracted the disease were admired and respected. It was in this era that the illness was dubbed The White Plague. The disease was seen to cause 'good death.' This was because the ailing could arrange their affairs and leave everything 'in order.' This was possible because the disease progressed with the pace of a tortoise. Many of the noblewomen would make up their faces to appear pale; this was called the consumptive appearance and was greatly admired. The disease was considered to be the disease of the rich, particularly the artists. Off the fantasy, people continued to get sick and would suffer from the illness. The poor people were blamed for facilitating the spread of the disease. The public health officers put in place measures to curb the spread of the disease. The officers prohibited the people from spitting in public and the streets, taking care of the infants and children, and quarantine that separated the people from their sick loved ones. The people, however, failed to follow these rules. The disease, like a bushfire, encroached far and wide and mercilessly disrupted people's lives and finally took them. It was in this century, on 24 March 1882, that Robert Koch identified Mycobacterium tuberculosis from patients' sputa. He proved to the people who knew little to do with microorganisms. He injected the infected matter from the corpses infected with tuberculosis into rabbits. The rabbits then developed the disease. Koch studied all the manifestations of tuberculosis and concluded that they were all caused by Mycobacterium tuberculosis. In 1890 Robert Koch isolated tuberculin, a protein derived from the bacterium. He attempted to use the protein as a vaccine, but this was not successful. However, tuberculin could be used for the diagnosis of tuberculosis. The care for patients who were suffering from tuberculosis improved little by little as new therapies were being used. Physicians realized isolating the patients from the healthy population would control the spread of the disease. Rene Laennec developed the stethoscope, which he used for auscultation. The instrument was used in the diagnosis of the disease and to measure the extent of the damage that the disease had caused. They established sanatoriums and clinics where they would take care of the patients in the 19th century, and saw numerous developments that were made towards understanding tuberculosis. This paved the way for the formulation of the vaccine and the cure. The white plague continued to rage against the people. In 1901, it was mentioned as the most serious problem in Britain. The following year, a Royal Commission was formed and instructed to establish the relationship between animal tuberculosis and human tuberculosis. They were asked to determine if the diseases could be transmitted from humans to animals and vice versa.

In Europe, an international commission was formed to tackle the problem. Albert Calmette and Camille Guerin developed the first successful vaccine against tuberculosis. This is known as the Bacillus-Calmette Guerin (BCG) vaccine, and it's used up to the present. The doctors in the 20th century used different approaches in treating tuberculosis because they had much more insight than their predecessors. They used varied techniques to try and cure this malady. For instance, they used a technique known as pneumothorax plombage, which involved collapsing of one affected lung. This was done to allow the lung to rest and heal from the tubercles. The method had been used by soldiers who had received sword wounds that affected the lungs. In as much as it was not a medical cure, it had therapeutic effectiveness, and many patients underwent it. In 1944, three scientists discovered a bacterium that was the first effective antibiotic against Mycobacterium tuberculosis. This was Streptomyces griseus. This marked the beginning of the modern era of the tuberculosis revolution, although some scientists argue that the true revolution occurred in 1952. It was in this year that the first oral drug against Mycobacteria was discovered. Streptomycin reduced the number of deaths due to tuberculosis by 51%. However, the mortality due to tuberculosis in England and Wales had reduced by 90-95% even before the discovery of Streptomycin and BCG vaccine. This mycobactericidal drug was known as isoniazid. The drug was used up to the 1970s when rifampin was discovered. The drug not only reduced the number of new cases of tuberculosis but also reduced the duration of recovery. Streptomycin raised the hopes that TB could be eradicated. It was so effective that the medical personnel started believing that with vaccines and the mycobactericides, they could win the war against the disease. However, their hopes were terribly crashed in the 1980s when there was the discovery of not one but several drug resistance strains. In 1987, there was a major resurgence in the number of new cases. In that year the number of cases was 5000, in the year 2000, the cases had risen to 6300, and in 2005, the cases were about 7600. One may wonder why this was the state of affairs. Medical sociologists argued that drugs could cure the existing cases of the disease, but poverty and poor living conditions reinforced the propagation of this contagion. They also noted that some factors, such as poor diet contributed to the persistence of the illness. A poor diet not only slowed the recovery process but also rendered the healthy population vulnerable to this disease due to weakened immunity. Another factor that contributed to the persistence of this malady was the fact that the majority of the resources were channeled to dealing with the global pandemic of HIV/AIDS. Moreover, TB was one of the opportunistic infections that plagued people living with HIV. Today we are still dealing with TB. One may not notice the measures that are taken to prevent new infections of the disease because they have been very well incorporated in our daily lives. Perhaps they were meant to be always in place. Take, for instance, vaccination against the disease. The BCG vaccine is one of the first vaccines that everyone gets, especially in countries with a high rate of TB. It is given at birth, and this plays a very big role in preventing infant tuberculosis infections. Other methods include proper ventilation of rooms and vessels of public transport. As the saying goes, an ounce of prevention is worth a pound of cure. The patients of tuberculosis are advised to take their medicine as prescribed by the doctor. This is done to ensure full recovery and avoid mutation of Mycobacterium into a drug-resistant strain. They are also advised to cover their mouths while coughing and sneezing to avoid spreading the disease to their loved ones. A proper diet is crucial to the patients to fortify their immunity to fight against this disease. They are also advised to avoid public transport to avoid exposing the public to the disease. There are low chances of the disease being transmitted from domestic animals to man. However, this can happen, especially via milk. People are therefore advised to boil milk before using it. Tuberculosis may sound like a disease of the olden days, but it continues to afflict pain on many people in the world. Let us not forget that some people have drug-resistant strains; in 2017, there were 558,000 new cases of Drug-resistant TB. Until more effective drugs are discovered, they continue to rely on treatment-therapy. This therapy is all-rounded and is comprised of proper care, social support, and support from medical personnel. This way, the patients can live a better life even when having this disease. World Tuberculosis Day is observed every year on 24 March. This day is to remind us of a disease that has plagued human beings since time immemorial. A disease that has taken away so many lives and caused so much agony. A malady that has proven to be hard to conquer because as we evolve, so does it. It continues to challenge our scientific methods as well as our social systems. This day reminds us that in as much as we may not be suffering from this disease, some people are. They continue to fight against this lifelong enemy. We should, therefore, stand with them in that battle because we may be healthy today, but never safe from it. Let us, in our small way, support the sick, the scientists, and the doctors in their struggle and aim to have a TB-free world.

The Plague of Justinian

The Plague of Justinian happened during the reign of Justinian in the Byzantine Empire (Eastern Roman Empire). The plague was caused by *Yersinia pestis,* a bacterium which originated from Central China, according to genetic evidence. It then spread to other parts of the world, mainly to Eurasia and Africa. This mostly happened through land and sea trade. The disease wreaked havoc during outbreaks that happened occasionally. But the Plague of Justinian was the greatest of the pandemics; it took about 25-100 million lives. The Plague of Justinian originated in Egypt, particularly in Pelusium. Egypt was, in that period, the major producer of grain in the world. They exported the grain to Europe, Asia, and other parts of Africa. It spread North to Europe and East to Palestine, and from there spread to the ends of the known world. It always started from the coast and then proceeded to the mainland. The plague was spread by the ships that transported grains to other parts of the world. The ships harbored fleas and black rats, which were vectors of the bacterium. When the ships docked at the harbors, the rats and the fleas would enter the land, and so did the plague. In 542 A.D., the plague reached Constantinople, the capital of the Byzantine Empire. A ship from Europe was bringing in grains; unknown to the sailors, and the city dwellers, the ship was full of plague-infested fleas and rats. The disease struck the city before spreading to the rest of the empire. The plague lurked for another 225 years and ended in 750 AD. The citizens started complaining of symptoms of the plague a few days after the arrival of the accursed ships. On the first day of infection, the patient experienced a really high fever. However, the patient's temperatures were not very high when touched. This did not raise any alarm, but unfortunately, some people died within 24 hours. This was followed by a feeling of malaise, whereby the patients would feel very weak. The patients then developed buboes, large swellings in the groin area, armpits, sometimes behind the ears and thighs. The black swellings were very painful and would grow up to the size of an egg. They were a sure sign that one was suffering from the plague. Some people died from the pain of the buboes, and those who passed this phase would either go into a coma or delirium. Those that were delusional could not feel the pain that the disease inflicted upon them. They would walk around with no one to take care of them. Most of them died due to a lack of sustenance, while others did harmful things to themselves. These people became hysterical and were paranoid. They would shout that some spirits or demons were after them. Procopius, a historian who, at the time of the plague, lived in Constantinople, documented that the people in delusion would walk right into the sea and drown. Those that were in a coma would remain in this state for a long time. If they had someone to take care of them, they would be fed and cleaned in this state. If they had no one, they would die due to a lack of sustenance. The disease caused those in a coma to forget their friends and themselves if and when they woke up. Some patients had necrosis of the hand, making them unable to carry out their former duties. Most people died within 24 hours after contracting the plague or within a few days. The people struggled to understand the plague in order to control it, but this proved to be an arduous task. The main reason was that the plague was fast-acting, causing the death of the patient just a few days after contracting it. This left little time for the testing of the remedies or treatments that would work. The plague had no rhythm in occurrence, and therefore could not be attributed to any phenomenon. The majority of the Romans were Christians, and they attributed the plague to have been caused by a demon. Many of them claimed to have had a vision of a demon telling them that they were in the list of the people that were supposed to be reaped. Some of the patients claimed to have seen the demon immediately after they woke up. Some patients did not experience this. One can't help but wonder, is it that they really saw the demons, or was it just the delusion that came by with the plague? Some people blamed the plague on Justinian, the Emperor, saying that he was a demon that had inflicted the illness upon his people. Due to the unpredictability of the occurrence of the disease, some people believed that the disease was the wrath of the gods, which happened when the transgressions of the people were too much. The people tried different ways to avoid the plague and its consequent excruciating suffering and death. They tried calling out holy names when they thought they had been exposed to the disease. They would exorcise these demons. Others, full of fear, would not go out from their houses lest they would mingle with the people and catch the pestilence. Others would not allow their neighbors, friends, or strangers in their home. Once the plague struck individuals, they either sought treatment by medical personnel or used home remedies. The physicians back then trained at Alexandria for four years. They learned directly from the practitioners. They became conversant with the principles that Galen had taught. They learned to treat illnesses based on humorism, which depended on the balance of body fluids. If the patients had no access to the physician, they used home remedies. The treatment and home remedies were as good as the exorcism of demons; it did not help. The people continued to suffer the effects of the plague. Scientists believe that the Plague of Justinian occurred in all three forms of plague. It occurred as bubonic, pneumonic, and septicemic plague. Bubonic plague is characterized by painful black swellings. Pneumonic plague affects the respiratory system. It is mainly transmitted via droplets in the air released by an infected person while coughing, talking, or sneezing. Septicemic plague affects the circulatory and lymphatic system. It is transmitted via the bite of a flea. The virulence of the plague suggests that it was the three types of plague that had infested the people. The Justinian Plague is considered to be the first pandemic ever to hit the globe and also the most lethal. The people had never witnessed such a plague. It would attack mildly at first, then with so much enragement and then would cause death within just a few days. It affected all levels of society; the rulers, the soldiers, the civilians, the young and old alike. The disease also affected animals such as cats and dogs. The disease spread so fast, partly due to the quests of the Roman soldiers to conquer more territories. This was due to Justinian's dream of gaining Rome's lost glory. The soldiers spread the disease to other places. The quests did not stop despite the plague that was raging, and this worsened the situation. Princes and paupers were both infected by the plague. Justinian himself was infected, but he later recovered. Romans experienced a shortage of food during the plague. This was because the farmers were no longer able to cultivate the land. The lands were left to weed. The reserves of grain continued to diminish day by day. Most bakers stopped working due to fear of contracting the plague. The food-sellers at the market were also locked behind their doors in fear of coming down with the pestilence. Day by day, the food became scarcer. Even those who had food were locked behind their houses and would not welcome anyone into their houses. It was a time of great suffering. The death toll of the Justinian Plague remains unparalleled in history. It halved the population of Europe just within two years. In Constantinople, about 10,000 people died each day. The people buried the dead until the cemeteries became full. More deaths continued in the city, and people started digging trenches for the safe disposal of the bodies. The trenches too were overwhelmed by the numbers of the bodies. The people, in desperation, started using the fortified towers of the city to dispose of the bodies. They would open the roof of the towers and throw in the bodies. They would throw them haphazardly, and the bodies would pile on top of each other until the tower was filled. They used all of the towers, but the bodies were increasing daily. Safe disposal of the corpses became such a difficult task to deal with that the emperor had to disburse some money for this purpose. Families were tasked with the responsibility of burying their relatives. Everyone was required to wear a wrist-band containing their name and that of their family. This was to facilitate easy recognition of the family, and therefore fast disposal of the deceased. The people lived in grief and did not know when the hour of their demise was coming. They lived in utter anticipation. Eventually, 40% of the people living in Constantinople perished The plague affected the economy of the Roman Empire immensely. The people were impoverished as they could no longer carry out their normal duties. However, their emperor did not exempt them from paying taxes. On the contrary, he made the people pay their taxes and cater for their dead relatives; how thoughtless? This was because the Emperor was committed to the construction of some public buildings, such as churches. For instance, the Hagia Sophia was a church in the capital which was still undergoing construction during the plague. The people's lives were balancing on the scales, and they were struggling to have something to put in their mouths. Was it fair to tax them at all, left alone the compensation of their dead relatives' tax? This is the best definition of ambition clouding one's judgment. Trade was crippled by the plague. Fewer farmers worked, and therefore less grain was produced. This caused the price of grains to rise, but the amount of revenue was less. Some of the traders refrained from trading in an attempt to evade the plague. Some died from the plague while others were taking care of their sick relatives. Commodities were scarce because there was no one to supply them to the traders. This affected internal trade within the Roman Empire and with the outside world. The economy was almost collapsing. Politically, the Empire was losing part of its territory because the empire could not withstand external attacks. The Lombards attacked and occupied the Italian Peninsula. The Arabs were also encroaching the Roman provinces that were in Northern Africa and occupied them. The Roman army was frail at the time of the plague, and more soldiers were lost than could be replaced. Many people were sick, dying, or dead. The healthy people were not willing to join the army, due to fear of the pestilence. Moreover, the Emperor was burdening them with too much taxation, and few were willing to serve him willingly. The empire became smaller, but their problems only became bigger. The Plague of Justinian lasted for two years. By the end of it, it had taken so much from the people. It left them with very many challenges and very little to start rebuilding their lives. It would take centuries for Europe to regain their former numbers. The Roman Empire lost some of its territories for good. The Plague of Justinian highlights the despondency that a crisis could cause. Plague recurred, and there is a possibility that it could recur in the future. How armed are we to deal with *Yersinia pestis*? Would unaffected countries take advantage of the countries dealing with the crisis, or would they stand together to deal with it?

The Black Death

You may have heard about the infamous Black Death, also known as the Great Bubonic Plague, the Great Pestilence, or the Great Mortality. This pandemic mostly affected Asia and Europe. The Black Death was a Bubonic plague caused by *Yersinia pestis*. This is a gram-negative, rod-shaped bacterium. According to historians, *Yersinia pestis* laid in a remote lake in central Asia, until in 1338, when the lake was disturbed by forces of nature, the bacterium infected fleas. The fleas then bit black rats, which carried the bacterium in its bloodstream. This led to the outbreak of The Plague, which spread to China, India, and other countries in the Far East. It also spread towards Asia Minor, Persia, Syria, and Egypt. The plague heavily affected the Middle East. Cairo was hit by this disease several times. In the 1340s, people in Europe heard rumors about a great pestilence that had affected the East. In 1347, the Mongols, a group of people who had been conquering Asia, reached Kaffa. They were led by Kipchak Khan Jani Beg. Kaffa was a Genoese trading port, a fortified town. The Mongols attacked Kaffa for several days, but the town was well-equipped to withstand attacks since it bordered the sea. The Mongols had been affected by the plague during their travel and conquest towards the west. Many of their soldiers had died, and they were desperate to conquer and acquire this rich and powerful town. On the third day, the Mongols started to catapult dead bodies into the fortified city, believing that those who were inside would catch the plague through the breathing of poisoned air. This was the first recorded use of biological weapons in history. In an attempt to avoid the plague, the people threw the dead and rotten bodies into the water. It was too late; the plague was already in their town. Moreover, they contaminated their water with bacteria responsible for it. After several days, people within the walls started dying. The symptoms of the plague were at first similar to those of heavy flu, and it was not anything one would worry about. Unpleasant symptoms such as fever, chills, and vomiting then followed, and this rendered many people weak and bed-ridden. The horrific symptoms came later, and this included buboes and boils, hence the term Bubonic Plague. Buboes are swellings that occur around the armpits and groin and are painful. They occurred when *Yersinia pestis* was carried to the lymph nodes via the lymphatic system. Black boils used to swell to the size of an egg or much larger. They were excruciating, and they would grow bigger and bigger. Eventually, they would burst and ooze pus and blood, making the patient have a purging odor. At this stage, the patient would wait for their death. This disease was also transmitted via coming in contact with infected body fluids such as pus and blood. This exposed not only the family members who had not yet been infected, but also the physicians, priests, and other care givers. After some time, physicians and priests refused to treat the plague patients in an attempt to avoid this malady. The death toll increased daily, and this eventually left the people utterly devastated. The people who dwelled in Kaffa were of different religions, including Islam and Christianity. They thought that this disease was a punishment from the gods and started interceding for mercy and forgiveness. This plague affected the rich and the poor alike. Each passing day brought along with it more misery and a cloud of lingering sadness. The people became too depressed, and they started planning dinners together. They believed that being together would help prevent stress, and consequently, the malady. This only worsened the situation by increasing the chances of healthy people contracting the disease. During the time of crisis, fear tends to take the front seat in the conducting of the affairs. Things were not different back then. As the number of dead people increased, people began to panic, and some fled from the once great, but now accursed, town of Kaffa. Some people fled Kaffa by twelve ships to the port of Messina in Sicily. As the ship docked in the harbor, the people were astonished to see that most of the crew members were already dead. Those who were alive were literally the walking dead. They were not only weak, but they also had boils. Furthermore, they were vomiting; they had a fever and experienced all those signs that characterized the infamous plague that was rumored to be in the East. The people in Sicily had already heard about the agony that came along with this monstrosity, and they were in panic, so they sent the ship away. This seems like a very wise thing to do, but the truth is that it yielded nothing at all. The moment the people walked into the ship and interacted with the coughing patients, they contracted the disease; it was airborne! The ship also had black rats, which are the secondary vectors of the bacterium, *Yersinia pestis*. As the people were inspecting the ship, the rats had already made their way to the land. This was how the Black Death reached Europe in October 1347. The disease then spread to the rest of Europe mostly along trade routes and ports. By 1349, much of lower Europe had been affected by the disease and had witnessed its awful effects. This includes Spain, France, Britain, and Italy. By 1351, countries in Eastern Europe were facing the scourge. The disease was spreading so fast, faster than a wildfire. It was claiming lives, mercilessly. Whole families died, villages were almost wiped, and even towns suffered. The Black Death decimated the population of Europe. The population decreased by about 60% between 1346 and 1353. It was a time of immense grief due to the loss of loved ones. Death became a part of their somewhat normal lives. It was only a matter of days that one passed away after contracting the disease. People believed the disease was a punishment from God. People started repenting and asking God for mercy. Radical members of the church became flagellants. They would mortify their bodies and the bodies of other flagellants as a sign of seeking God's mercy. Some lost faith in the church as the prayers didn't solve the plague. It was a time of great fear because some people didn't know how long it would be before the plague took their lives. People became poorer because when the disease affected them, they could no longer carry out their economic duties. The farmers could no longer farm; the traders could no longer trade; the teachers could no longer teach, and so on. Food became scarce, and people became malnourished. In the marketplaces, the price of things drastically rose because almost everything was scarce. In the 14th century, so many sheep had died that Europe was experiencing a drastic shortage of wool, hence clothing. This period devastated the social institutions, but mostly, religion and family. The Black Death greatly weakened the people due to several reasons. First, the medical knowledge in the 13th century was very scarce. People could barely deal with diseases such as common cold; therefore, Bubonic Plague was hard to conquer. They did not know what caused the disease. Some people suggested wrath from gods, others miasma, noxious air, but no one knew the real cause. *Yersinia pestis* was discovered in the 19th century. Physicians tried as much as they could to cure this malady. Here are some of the methods that were used. Patients were instructed to drink their urine. It may seem very strange and disgusting in our age, but we have to understand that the doctors were acting according to the teachings of Hippocrates. Hippocrates taught about the balance of humor in the body, which brought about health and imbalance brought about illness. Urine was believed to have a good balance of the humor and that drinking or bathing in it would restore health. The physicians also thought that the disease caused one to have bad blood. They, therefore, drained the blood by using leeches, which sucked the patients, or they would let the blood drain. They believed that by so doing, they would not only drain corrupted blood but also restore the balance of humor hence health. Treacle was used to treat the sick. It is a sticky substance made from sugar that had been left to be ready for at least 10 years. It was believed to harbor fungi and other organisms necessary to fight and eliminate the corruption of the body. Another method used was the live cock method. The cock was used to relieve the boils. Quarantine was a method that was discovered much later. It involved making the sick person stay away from those who are well. This way, the sick were taken care of while leaving the healthy people at minimal risk. Doctors made themselves protective clothing. They had a face mask that had a beak-like projection, which was believed to filter out the miasma. It had glass openings for the eyes. The overall also protected the doctor from the fluids of the infected patient. It is believed that quarantining sick patients led to the steady decline of the deaths of patients suffering from the Black Death and the number of new cases. The Black Death is a clear illustration of how the lack of knowledge can cost us lives, and it can cause suffering and great loss. It also shows how superstition can be a challenge to effective disaster management. This plague is considered a turning point in history because Europe only recovered from it about 150 years later. This was one of the greatest pestilences in history, may we learn from it.

The Great Plague of Marseille

The Great Plague of Marseille was a pandemic that hit different parts of the world, especially the Middle East and North Africa. Our focus will be on the city of Marseille, which faced the pandemic and had to battle with this plague, which was the last of its kind. Marseille is a port in southern France. The city is as old as a rock because it was established in 600BC as the Greek colony of Massalia. From Massalia, its name was coined. It was initially populated by Greeks. Marseille was politically formidable, and in 218 BC, the city-state helped the Roman Empire in the battle against Carthage. It was a great city that was once an early center of Christianity in Western Europe. The city has seen prosperity as well as downfall. Marseille has ruled, she has been seized and once again rose, several times. The city has contributed quite a lot to France as a nation. For instance, it was the focal point of the French Revolution, which changed the country's politics for good. Furthermore, the French National Anthem, La Marseillaise, originated from this remarkable city. It has also witnessed some significant setbacks, the greatest of which is the Great Plague of Marseille. The Great Plague of Marseille reached the city port in 1720. It arrived in a merchant ship known as Grand-Saint-Antoine. The vessel is said to have departed from the port of Sidon, Lebanon, but had previously docked at Tripoli, Smyrna, and Cyprus. The ship actually picked up the plague from Cyprus. One of the crew members, a Turkish man, was the first to be infected and died within a short period. The disease spread to other crew members very fast, and the ship's surgeon was not spared. Devastated by the disease, the crew members tried to dock at Livorno, Italy, but the Italians denied them entry. Slowly but surely, the crew members had to await arrival back home at Marseille. The crew members were immediately placed under quarantine at the Lazarets that had been put in place for this purpose. The plague has been named 'Great,' and this may be considered as a misnomer because its effects were far from great. They were debilitating, deleterious, and traumatic. It took not only time but also courage and the sheer willingness of the inhabitants of Marseille and other parts of France to recover from this devastating pandemic. The pestilence was the bubonic plague which had manifested itself for the first time during the Black Death. The Black Death had devastated Eurasia in the 14th century. The plague occurred several times after the Black Death, so it was not a new thing to the people of Marseille. The city dwellers had witnessed other outbreaks in the city. They had risen to the occasion and put in place measures to contain infectious diseases and prevent the occurrence of additional explosions. At the end of a plague that struck the city in 1580, the people decided to form a sanitation board. The members of this board were to be picked from the city council and a group of doctors. The board's first duty was to ensure that the city was clean at all times, as this would prevent diseases from attacking the dwellers. They would also protect the city from exterior vulnerabilities to do with disease. Furthermore, the board was to improve health-related infrastructure; in fact, the first public hospital in Marseille was built following the recommendation of the committee. The hospital was well-equipped with doctors and nurses. The people of Marseille realized that plagues were usually an opportunity for the spread of propaganda to do with the disease afflicting the people. For this reason, the board accredited doctors who would be relied on to spread accurate information in case of a pestilence. This would play a significant role in the prevention and control of diseases. Quarantine was yet another system that the people of Marseille used in an attempt to ward off diseases. They used a 3-tier quarantine system, which proved efficient in the prevention of disease outbreaks in the city. The system mainly focused on monitoring ships and its crew members since merchant ships were the main method in which these diseases were being transmitted from one place to another. In the first tier, some members of the sanitation board observed crew members, passengers, and cargo for any signs of disease. They also inquired about the ports and cities where the ship landed while counterchecking it to a list of cities rumored to be afflicted with any disease. If people in the vessel tested negative for symptoms and had not landed at any city of suspicion, they were allowed into the city. Otherwise, the ship had to undergo quarantine in a lazaret for at least 18 days. A lazaret was an isolated island, a mainland building, or a ship that was permanently anchored where marine travelers would be isolated for some time. The lazarets were well-ventilated for the efficient release of miasmas that caused the disease. The facilities were near the sea to ensure an excessive supply of water for thorough and frequent cleaning. A ship would proceed to the second tier if none of the members aboard had the symptoms of a disease even though they entered a city or port rumored to be plagued by a particular disease. If they did not develop the signs and symptoms of illness within 18 days, they were allowed to enter the city. If people developed the symptoms, they entered the third tier where the people were treated of their various ailments until they were declared safe to interact with other people without the risk of infecting them. The ship that brought with it the Great Plague of Marseille passed on the disease despite all these measures. One could only ponder how that could happen. The ship that carried the pestilence arrived in March 1720. From then on, the disease spread slowly from one person to another. In May, the effects of the disease, though still minute by then, were felt when two women died from the bubonic plague. Little did the inhabitants of Marseille know that the situation would only aggravate. The disease was caused by a bacterium known as *Yersinia pestis*, whose primary vector is fleas. The fleas may bite humans and transmit the bacterium to the human body. They may also bite rats and spread the bacterium to the bloodstream of rats, which then bite human beings. The signs and symptoms that afflicted the inhabitants of Marseille were excruciating, and they prevented them from carrying out their day to day activities. They would first experience flu-like symptoms, which included fever, headaches, and vomiting. The symptoms would then progress and become more and more dangerous. The patient would develop buboes around the groin and armpit. This was due to the fact that the bacteria divided around the lymph nodes and caused black swellings, which were the hallmark of this infamous malady. The victim would also suffer painful muscle spasms, bloody vomiting, and gangrene. Their fever became higher, and the patient would fall into a coma and finally die. The disease was highly contagious because it could affect families and wipe them out. Even after the infected person died, the contagion lived on, ready to infect anyone who would come into contact with the body. The Sanitation board noticed this and advised that if a family had been wiped out, their houses should be sealed to avoid contamination. The malady caused untold suffering, grief as well as terror among the inhabitants of Marseille. There were several hospitals in the city which started admitting people who were afflicted with the plague. The doctors had a hard time coming up with a cure for this plague. Some recommended herbal medicine and improved diet. Other doctors thought that the swellings could be used as a port to release noxious humor that caused the disease. Some doctors also lit fires in the wards to ward off noxious miasmas released by the patients. The physicians tried to combat this disease to no avail. More people came to the hospitals, but no cure had been found, and people continued to die. The hospitals were overwhelmed, the staff overworked, and the doctors despaired. People started to panic because their only hope was in their health system whose work was yielding no fruits during the crisis. The disease affected all, young and old, poor, and rich. It disrupted the lives of millions of people, caused immense suffering and death. In Marseille, the hospital infirmaries could not hold such a massive amount of bodies. More and more corpses kept coming in; in desperation, some of the bodies were thrown in the streets. This act did no good in as much as prevention of the disease was concerned. The members of the sanitation board, therefore, ordered for the proper disposal of the deceased by at least digging mass graves. In the city, about 1000 people died each day. As the situation worsened, it was more cumbersome to dig graves for the increasing number of corpses. Those who dug it were at risk of contracting the lethal illness. As necessity is the mother of invention, Le Mur de Peste was constructed around this period. Le Mur de Peste - the Wall of Pestilence - was a wall 2 meters high and 70 cm thick. Bodies of those whose death was caused by the plague were thrown beyond the wall. This practice was easier, faster, and less risky compared to the digging of graves. Nonetheless, the disease continued spreading among the people. The situation in Marseille worsened daily. The destruction was so profound that other cities forbade their inhabitants from having contact with anyone from Marseille. Failure to follow these instructions led to heavy punishment. Aix is one of the cities that passed this sort of legislation. The plague continued to bug the inhabitants, causing misery and grief. It also spread to other parts of the country, such as Aix, Toulon, and Arles. The plague affected the city port of Marseille profoundly. It has always been remembered as one of the worst tragedies to ever happen to the city. It enervated the city economically, politically, and socially. The inhabitants of Marseille were used to having control over situations. They were good planners who had earlier been able to avoid and contain most diseases. They had what by the standards of that time seemed to be the best health system, yet the plague gave them a resounding blow. This plague demeaned them and devitalized their spirit. The people who had earlier on, been a subject of admiration were now to be avoided at all costs. It made most of them resentful. The city-dwellers were all at risk of contracting the contagion that was *Yersinia pestis*. They were facing the loss of friends, peers, families, and their leaders. The loss caused depression and untold misery. Where there is a crisis, there is fear. The inhabitants of

Marseille did not escape this vice. Overwhelmed by its power, over 10% of the inhabitants fled from the city to avoid the seething wrath of the plague. Their city that was once magnificent and clean was littered with bodies throughout the streets. This was not a pleasant sight. Trade, which was the main economic activity of the people of Marseille, was impossible during this plague that lasted for about two years. The pestilence weakened the city's position as far as the economy was concerned. The people could no longer farm; they could no longer take part in local trade within the city or international trade. The fishermen could not fish. The artists could not make their artifacts, let alone sell them. It was a time of economic dormancy that hit the people hard. Many people used most of their resources in the treatment of their sick relatives, and this sapped them financially. Most importantly, there was a shortage of food within the city due to the plague. The people incited each other to riot due to the numerous troubles they were going through and because, deeply engrained in their souls was the fear of dying. As the French say, petit a petit, little by little, the plague started dying out. By the spring of 1721, the death toll had reduced to about one person per day. By the winter of 1722, the plague died out, and there was no longer cause for despair. It was the last of the outbreaks of Bubonic plague in Europe. Bubonic plague is infamous for being the reaper of souls in the olden days, and this time was no exception. It caused death after all the misery that the patient had gone through in the course of the illness. Once one had contracted the disease, it was only a matter of days until they would leave the land of the living. By the time the plague was dying out in 1722, the plague had claimed half of the population of Marseille. It did not spare other cities, Aix and Arles lost 25% of their population each. Toulon did not escape the grim reaper, which claimed more than 50% of her inhabitants. The plague claimed, in total, about one-third of France's population. Such is the power of a plague; it strips a nation of its numbers, power, and pride. Finally, the plague died during the winter of 1722. Scientists speculated that the causative agents could not survive the cold. The deaths dropped steadily, and so did the new cases of the disease. The disease hit the city so hard that many thought that Marseille would take ages to recover. However, the inhabitants of this city worked so hard and recovered in a short period that historians are astonished to date. The trade became even more established and reached new regions such as Latin America and the West Indies. The population was reaching the pre-plague numbers by 1765. Generally, things were not so bad for the city. Despite the lack of solid knowledge on what caused the plague, the physicians and the Sanitary Board put up measures to prevent such a pestilence from reoccurring. Quarantine methods became more strict, and the people who were checking the ships became more careful. The Lazaret d'Arenc, a water-side building, was established by the royal government to increase the city's defense against the plague. It was a double line of fifteen-foot walls ringed. The walls were pierced on the sides facing the water to permit the offloading of cargo. The Great Plague of Marseille had a couple of lessons in store for the people of Marseille and also to the modern world. The plague showed the importance of fomes in the transmission of disease-causing microorganisms, how so? Despite the people's measures to quarantine the ship that carried the plague, fomes, which was mainly the commodities of trade, spread the disease far and wide. This lesson has been taken into consideration in recent outbreaks of plagues whereby commodities are not bought from the afflicted areas. The plague also showed that despite the human measures put in place to prevent disaster, it may still strike and cause immense destruction to human beings. This lesson can be applied to crises, and it can prevent the blame-game and hatred that comes along with crises. It also shows the importance of the ages-old quarantine method in the containing of contagions and other outbreaks. The bubonic plague also showed the importance of health services in the time of epidemics. In as much as they were unable to provide a solution to the looming disease, they gave hope to the despairing community and took care of the sick. They also played a great role in trying to explain the cause of the illness to the people, and this calmed their fears a bit. They gave directives on what to be done during the crises. For instance, how to dispose of the bodies of the deceased safely. This convinced the people that the health services were still working towards improving the situation even though things were getting out of hand. The people of Marseille showed us how people could turn their situation after facing a crisis for their own good. The people of Marseille thrived despite the devastating toll that the plague had taken on each sector of the city. It shows us that instead of wallowing in self-pity and longing for the lost, we can create anew, bigger, and better. Crises have the power of bringing out the true character of human beings. The neighbors of Marseille turned a cold shoulder to the people when they needed help most. The inhabitants of this city needed more physicians, food supply, and other gestures of support from their neighbors. However, all they got from them was rejection and abandonment. This opened the people's eyes to the fact that they had to be independent in the management of crisis such that they could face and deal with it, with or without external help. In my opinion, this lesson was one of the driving forces for the city to become a better one. May we not forget that despite the force that the disease may hit the world with, we can always recover. We can re-establish our world to be a better place than it was before. Everyone should use their time and resources productively. This way, we can learn ways in which we can recover socially, economically as well as politically. May the Great Plague of Marseille remind us that we have a purpose to survive the pandemic and rebuild.

Cholera Pandemic

Cholera is an acute diarrheal disease which is caused by a bacterium called *Vibrio cholera*. The disease has existed for a long time. The origin of the disease is said to be Ganges, India. Before the 19th century, several outbreaks had occurred in India. Up to date, the disease continues to be a threat to some communities where the disease is endemic. This term means that the disease is found locally in the community, and active transmission takes place, and no infection comes from outside the area. It is important to note that an outbreak can occur in an area that is endemic or not. Cholera outbreaks are usually very severe and cost many lives. *Vibrio cholera* is a microorganism that tends to survive in warm places, especially in water. There are many strains or serogroups of the bacterium. However, only two have been seen to cause outbreaks. These are O1 and O139. *Vibrio cholera* O1 has been the cause of all recent cholera outbreaks, while O139 only caused epidemics in the past. Moreover, the strain O139 has not yet been identified outside Asia. Both serogroups cause the same illness, cholera. There is absolutely no difference in the manifestations of the strain when they infect the human body. Cholera is a very virulent disease that affects both children and adults. When one is infected, they may show symptoms within hours or after a few days. The patients develop smelly, whitish diarrhea. Most patients describe it as rice-water diarrhea. It is whitish due to the disruption of mucous membranes along the digestive tract by the bacteria. The diarrheal fluid volume varies from 10-18 liters depending on the severity of the illness. The patients also vomit a lot. The vomit, coupled with diarrhea, causes dehydration and imbalance of electrolytes within the body, making cholera a deadly disease. Dehydration also causes the skin to lose elasticity, making it wrinkled and the mucous membranes to be dry. Moreover, patients become very thirsty. Furthermore, severe dehydration causes the patient to have low blood pressure, which interferes with the normal functioning of the body. The heart rate becomes rapid in an attempt to make up for low blood pressure. They experience excruciating muscle cramps as well as fatigue. Patients release little or no urine as a result of severe water loss via diarrhea and throwing up. In extreme cases, patients may experience septic shock, seizures, or death. There have been seven cholera pandemics between the 19th and 20th centuries. The first cholera pandemic occurred between 1817 and 1824 in Calcutta. That is why it is also known as the first Asiatic cholera pandemic. It then spread to South East Asia, the Middle East, Eastern Africa, as well as the Mediterranean coast. The disease affected almost every country in Asia. It claimed hundreds of thousands of lives. It is crucial to understand that even before this pandemic, the disease had been endemic in the area in the lower Ganges River. From here, it used to spread to the rest of India, and outbreaks would occur. The spread of the disease was facilitated by the pilgrims who visited the Ganges, and obviously carried the bacteria to other places. Contaminated rice from the Ganges that was sold to other parts of India also played a significant role in the spread of the pestilence. The disease spread so fast, and by 1818, there was an epidemic at Bombay, and by 1830 it was already in Thailand. By 1821, China had already reported many cases of the malady. Japan experienced it by 1822. One may wonder why the disease was spreading so fast. We have to understand that cholera is a water-borne disease. This means that the causative agent can live in water, and the disease is, therefore, mainly transmitted via contaminated water. Contaminated food also plays a massive role in the transmission of the contagion. Raw and undercooked shellfish, fresh fruits, and vegetables have been highlighted as some of the main fomites of the bacterium. When a human being gets infected with cholera, they release the bacteria in their stool. This can happen whether or not the patient has symptoms. The stool is a potential contaminant of the water sources around. If the bacteria get to the water source, many people become infected, and this usually ends up in an outbreak. The living conditions during the first cholera pandemic were poor. The people were living in congested rooms. Water sources were not well protected, and that is why the disease tended to attack the entire communities. The British troops traveling from India spread cholera to the Persian Gulf. From the Gulf, it made its way to Turkey, southern Russia, and Syria. The first cholera pandemic affected a vast area and equally claimed so many lives. On the island of Java alone, it claimed 100,000 lives. In British India, 1.5 million people died from this disease while in the Thai capital city, Bangkok, 30,000 lives were lost. Undoubtedly, the death toll was high. The disease was and is still so deadly because the bacterium releases toxins in the body. The toxins are toxic to the body. In an attempt to flush out the hazardous toxins, the body releases too much water. The patient loses considerable amounts of water via diarrhea and vomit. This leaves the body dehydrated, with low blood pressure and a rapid heartbeat, perfect conditions for death to occur. The first cholera pandemic died out in 1824. During winter, the virus could not survive in the frigid weather. The people could heave a sigh of relief but not for long. The disease would recur not once but severally, as pandemics. It continues to plague the modern world, especially in areas with poor sanitation. The second cholera pandemic started two years after the end of the first pandemic. It happened between 1826 and 1837, a total of eleven years. The second pandemic was more horrific than the first one. It killed swiftly; it took many lives in a short time. The origin of these pandemics remains a subject of debate. Some scientists argue that the first cholera pandemic lingered in some areas such as the Philippines and Indonesia, and it just spread to other parts. Others say that the second cholera pandemic was independent of the first. It originated from the Ganges, just like the first and spread out. This pandemic spread far more extensively than the first. The second cholera pandemic afflicted Asia and spread along trade routes. It afflicted the whole of India, then spread to China by 1826, Iran by 1829, and Japan by 1831. The pestilence also spread across Europe and Continental America. In August 1831, during the invasion of Moscow, cholera infiltrated Russia, and consequently, the rest of Europe. By 1831, cholera plagued Russia in a significant way. It affected everyone everywhere in villages, towns, and cities. In Warsaw, 4,740 people fell ill, and 2,530 died from the disease. Russia reported a total of 100,000 deaths. The pestilence was spreading very fast. During the Polish-Russian war that took place between 1830 and 1831, the Russian soldiers transmitted the disease without their knowledge to Polish soldiers. The Russian soldiers also spread the sickness to East Prussia. As a result, several governments closed their borders to Russians in an attempt to avoid the disease. The people dreaded the disease due to the corporal suffering and death it caused. Governments started creating and enforcing anti-cholera laws to curb the spread of the disease. It is documented that there were several riots in Russia against the new regulations in 1831. In an attempt to protect her people, the British government ordered mandatory quarantine for all the ships that came from Russia to British ports. The board of health advised the people to eliminate all kinds of filth from their homes by burning the trash. They urged the people to do away with anything that could bring noxious air, miasma. They believed that miasma was the cause of the pandemic. For one to avoid the disease, they had to do away with noxious air. Rags, old newspapers, old clothing, and furniture were cleansed using boiled water and lime. Houses were to have fresh air. The board also called for general hygiene. Some British doctors observed the disease at St Petersburg. They documented the signs and symptoms of the disease, which they made known to the public as a precaution. The signs included giddiness, cramps beginning at the tips of the fingers and toes, vomiting, diarrhea, and sinking of the eyes in the sockets. They also recorded that the complexion of the victim would change to purple, blue, leaden, or black, depending on the severity of the attack. The toes would reduce in size, the skin would be stone-cold, and the respiration would be quick and irregular. The people were urged to report the cases as soon as one developed the signs. In December 1931, the pestilence reached Great Britain when a passenger ship from the Baltic docked in Sunderland. The disease spread to the rest of the country. Compared to other nations, the disease affected Britain mildly because they had improved their hygiene as a precaution. In London, 6,536 victims died due to cholera, while in Paris, 20,000 were lost. This shows the importance of preparedness during a pandemic. The pandemic had already reached America by 1832. It caused dread in Quebec and Ontario, Canada. It caused agony in Detroit and New York City in the USA. As if the second cholera pandemic had not caused enough trouble, the third cholera pandemic happened. The pandemic, just like the first two, started in the Ganges Delta and spread to the four corners of the globe. This time, the malady was way more virulent than the first two times. It caused the highest fatalities in the 19th century. In the vast land of Russia, more than one million people perished. The disease caused the death of 10,000 people in London alone, and a total of 23,000 people in Great Britain. John Snow, the Father of Modern Epidemiology, identified the source of the disease in the area where he was working. He mapped out the cases of cholera in Soho, where he was working and realized that contaminated water from a public water source was the cause of the disease. He instructed the closure of the plagued water pump. This led to an immediate decline in new cases. In as much as the third cholera pandemic caused so much loss, it was an eye-opener to the public on how to contain the disease in case of future attacks. The USA and Great Britain were some of the countries that improved water and sanitation, especially in cities. This gave them an upper hand while dealing with future cholera pandemics. The fourth cholera pandemic occurred in 1863-1875, while the fifth occurred between 1881 and 1896. For most parts of the world, the outbreaks were less severe compared to those that happened prior. The virulence of the disease, as well as the viciousness of the symptoms, were way less terrific. However, some countries suffered deadly outbreaks and lost a massive chunk of their population. Take, for instance, in Hungary, the country lost 190,000 who perished due to cholera outbreak between 1872 and 1873. In Hamburg, Germany, 1.5% of the population was lost during the fifth cholera outbreak. The sixth cholera pandemic was a molly pestilence which affected less area compared to the other pandemics. Western Europe and North America were not affected by the pandemic. This was because of the advances these areas had made in the public health sector. Water and sanitation were in proper condition in these places, making them safe from cholera. The disease savaged India, Africa, the Middle East, and Russia, which presented perfect conditions for the disease to thrive. The pandemic started in 1899. It progressed to its peak, which was in 1918 and 1919. At its peak, it caused massive deaths, especially in India, where it claimed more than half a million lives. It then started dissipating slowly but surely. By 1923, cholera had disappeared. It may be surprising to some people that we are in the course of the seventh cholera pandemic. This pandemic started in 1961. Unlike the other pandemics, it originated from Indonesia and spread out to the rest of the world. It spread throughout Asia and was reported in Africa in 1971. It took a heavy toll on Africa due to inadequate water supply and sanitation. It claimed many lives. Due to the slow action in the improvement of water supply systems and the provision of clean water, the disease lingered longer in the continent than in other affected areas. In 1990, 90% of all the cases that the World Health Organization recorded were from Africa. In 1991, the unexpected happened in South America. Cholera resurged after 100 years of the sub-continent being cholera-free. It was first observed in Peru, where it claimed 3,000 lives in 1991. It then spread to Chile, Colombia, then Central America, and Mexico. Though the current pandemic has already affected about 120 countries, the disease hovers above the less-developed and impoverished countries. These nations continue to bear the yoke of devastating outbreaks. Zimbabwe suffered an outbreak that affected about 97,000 people and took 4,250 lives in 2009. The Haiti outbreak of 2011, which followed the massive Haiti earthquake, affected half a million people. In 2017, Yemen and Somalia lost 2,000 people to cholera outbreaks. Judging by the number of lives that cholera has cost in the past and present, it is accurate to say that cholera is life-threatening. The threat of the disease is most especially felt in the less-developed world where the disease kills swiftly due to the lack of fast and efficient medical care. The disease spreads fast in these areas due to poor water and sanitation. Treating cholera is a straight-forward process of rehydrating the body and killing the bacteria in the body. Eighty-five percent of the cases of cholera can be treated using oral rehydration solution. However, severe cases require the intravenous infusion of liquids as well as antibiotics to combat the bacterium. Every year, about 1.3 to 4 million cases of cholera are reported. Of these, 23,000 to 143,000 people die from this disease. These high values show the gravity of the situation as per now. It is still surprising how some parts of the world have steered clear of this disease while it continues to plague others. The World Health Organization set up measures to curb the current cholera pandemic in 2017. The strategies outlined some measures to prevent the outbreak of the disease. The first and most potent weapon in the battle against this pestilence is proper sanitation and the provision of clean water. Moreover, the WHO insists on the practice of good food hygiene. Food should be appropriately cleaned before eating or preparation. It should also be well cooked. Health education to the community members is also an essential measure in combating the disease. The community should be well conversant with proper hygiene measures. They should wash their hands regularly with soap and clean running water. They should only consume pure and safe drinking water.

The WHO also approved a safe oral vaccine that can be used to protect people against the disease. However, the organization discourages the routine use of antibiotics because they play no role in controlling the spread of the disease but rather increases antimicrobial resistance. In my opinion, cholera is one of the most straightforward diseases to deal with. Once clean and safe water is sufficient, the mountain of the problem becomes a walkover. Proper sanitation ensures that the people have clean water supply, and the source is protected from contamination. The world can beat cholera better than it did with guinea worm disease. However, this requires proper strategizing and even better implementation of the strategy. Moreover, plans should be put in place in case of the reemergence of the bacteria. We can achieve the vision of a cholera free world in 3 simple steps which are; do, teach, and help. Do what should be done to prevent the spread of the disease and to promote health. Be an excellent teacher and spread health education concerning cholera. Step by step, little by little, we will reduce the cases of cholera and finally eradicate it.

Measles

Measles has been referred to as an ancient disease that doesn't affect the modern world. Make no mistake, in 2019, the disease resurged in America where there were more than 700 cases in 22 states. Now it may be a reason for us to take caution. It was also a nightmare in the first half of the 20th century when it caused many deaths and hospitalization. Let us try and understand this disease of the olden days, its pathology, cure, and most importantly, how we can prevent it. Measles, also known as rubeola, red measles or English measles, is an acute viral infection. It is caused by the measles virus, which is also known as rubeola virus. The virus is single-stranded and enveloped. This disease is airborne. The virus is usually spread by droplets when an infected person coughs, sneezes, or talks. It can also be transmitted by direct contact with the body fluids of an infected person, especially those from their respiratory tract. The virus attaches to the mucosal lining of the respiratory system and starts attacking the victim's body. Measles virus is the most contagious virus, and it remains infective in the airspace up to one hour after exhalation by the sick person. It infects up to 90% of the people surrounding the ailing person, making it very difficult to control. Several factors make one susceptible to infection by the virus. First, if one is immuno-compromised in any way, they become vulnerable to measles infection. Take, for instance, when one is immuno-deficient because they are battling a disease that weakens the immune system, they catch the virus very easily. These diseases include cancer and HIV/AIDS, among others. One may also be susceptible if they are immuno-suppressed; this happens when one's immunity has been instructed by the body to tolerate some things that may otherwise be deemed as foreign. This phenomenon occurs when one has received an organ transplant or is undergoing corticosteroid therapy. In such cases, one can easily be put down by this virus because after infection takes place, their bodies can't fight off the illness, and it ends up wreaking destruction in their bodies. When one is unvaccinated, they get easily infected. The vulnerability also applies to those who often travel internationally as well as those with a deficiency of Vitamin A. The incubation period of the virus is up to 14 days. This means that the virus can be transmitted unknowingly before the signs and symptoms occur. The signs are, at first, typical to a viral infection. A fever of about 40 degrees Celsius is the very first symptom that a measles patient will experience. This is followed by dry cough, runny nose, sore throat, and croup. At this point, the patient may mistake measles for the flu, and this is what makes the blow given by the disease really tough. The eyes then appear red due to conjunctivitis, the inflammation of the conjunctiva. This may be the reason why the condition is also known as red measles. Koplik's spots then develop in the mouth. These are white spots which have bluish-white centers and are found opposite the molars. The tell-tale sign then appears, a skin rash with huge, flat blotches that run into one another. There are also complications that come about as a result of measles. They occur due to the immuno-suppression as a result of the measles virus in the body. The most common complication caused by measles is the infection of the middle ear. The infection is mostly bacterial infection. In severe cases, it may cause loss of hearing. Measles also causes pneumonia, which may be viral or secondary bacterial. Pneumonia associated with measles is a significant cause of death. Another serious complication that occurs is known as encephalitis. Encephalitis is the inflammation of the brain and is quite common when one has viral infections. The problem with measles is that encephalitis may occur in the course of the illness or after one has been cured of measles. This makes it hard to detect, and it may cause severe cognitive problems, and eventually, it may cause death. Measles could be lethal to unborn babies as the disease could cause preterm labor. Moreover, it causes low birth weight and maternal mortality. Less commonly, measles cause seizures and blindness. Measles is a very ancient disease because it was mentioned as early as the 9th

Century BC by Rhazes, a Persian physician. He similarly describes the disease as smallpox, although he said it was worse than smallpox. Considering that the virus keeps on mutating, the physician had done an impeccable job in recording the symptoms of the illness. The virus may have evolved from rinderpest in cattle as a zoonotic disease. In China, early doctors say that the disease has been there since time immemorial, although there are high chances that they were confusing this malady with smallpox or chickenpox. The disease continued to cause enormous harm to human lives. Physicians in England and Spain thought that the disease miasmas or vapors that emerged from the ground caused the pestilence. This was a great misconception because failure to note that the disease could be transmitted from one person to another increased the spread due to lack of precautions. The condition was remotely understood until 1757 when John Homes established that an infectious agent was the cause of the disease. The disease affected many people around the globe. For instance, in 1529, it hit Cuba very hard. There was an outbreak that wiped out two-thirds of the population. This suggests that the people were being exposed to the virus for the first time. That is why they succumbed, despite having survived a smallpox epidemic that had happened before this. In 1531, the disease caused the death of half of the population of Honduras. The pestilence caused utter despondency in Mexico and the Inca civilization. Measles continued to infect human beings, causing utter agony and bringing death to the young and old alike. In the USA, it was reported for the first time in 1765. It killed around 6,000 people per year, while 48,000 people were hospitalized. Physicians strived to cure it or to treat its symptoms with varying degrees of success. It influenced human life so much that in the first half of the 20th century, it was considered a natural, universal thing that happens at a point in every child's life. Outbreaks of measles continued to occur time and time again in different parts of the world. In the 1800s, measles was considered to be endemic to

England. It was also afflicting people in Spain and the rest of the Old World. It then spread widely to the New World, as access to the world increased, so did the chances of the introduction of this disease to virgin populations. The disease continued to afflict human beings and also influenced the culture and lifestyle of the people. In the first half of the 20th century, the disease was prevalent in the world. It affected hundreds of thousands of people around the globe and killed tens of thousands. Measles continued to devastate the people physically because of their disrupting symptoms, and they could not work or continue with their normal activities. In 1915, the death toll due to the disease in the USA was the highest in the 20th century, at 14,000 deaths. Today, we know of the vaccine against measles that almost every child acquires. In 2015, 85% of the population of the children in the world were vaccinated against measles. One may wonder why the vaccine is administered at 9-15 months as opposed to at birth, considering the frustration caused by this malady. We have to understand that nature has provided a natural way for the child to protect his/herself against measles; how so? Antibodies, specifically, IgG, are transmitted from the mother to the fetus. The levels remain above protective levels up to one year after birth, amazing, right? After this, the children are usually administered the measles vaccine in combination with vaccines against Mumps and Rubella. It is collectively known as MMR. How was the vaccine developed? What were the problems encountered? There was an outbreak of measles in a school in Massachusetts in 1954. Two doctors, John F Enders and Thomas C Peebles, visited the school and collected blood samples from several ill students. They aimed to isolate the measles virus from the samples and develop a vaccine against the disease. They successfully isolated the virus from the blood sample of 13-year-old David Edmondston. They then developed the Edmonston B-strain measles virus vaccine. The vaccine, however, proved to be too intense for some people. These people developed the symptoms of the disease because their bodies could not fight the virus and develop the immunity required against the disease. This phenomenon made some people paranoid about the vaccines. In 1971, Maurice Hilleman & Co. came up with the MMR vaccine, which was effective against mumps, measles, and rubella. The vaccine has been further in some places in the world to include the Varicella zoster virus, commonly known as chickenpox. This enhanced vaccine is known as MMRV The vaccine was, at first, not well received because people had 'bigger problems.' For instance, poor Americans found the vaccine too costly. It cost 10$ (about 80$ today), and the people had other matters to take care of. They were struggling to make ends meet. People started spreading rumors that the measles vaccine could be deadly in an attempt to make it unpopular. However, the vaccine prevented so many deaths each year. It proved so effective that measles death became so rare, and most people started believing that measles could not kill. In 1978, the CDC (Center for Disease Control and Prevention) set a goal to eliminate measles by 1982. This goal was, however, not met. Despite this setback, the disease rate dropped dramatically, and by 1981, only 20% of the cases in the pre-vaccine era were still prevailing. This drastic drop shone a ray of hope. In 1989, there were measles outbreaks in America, especially in schools. The outbreaks affected children who had initially received the vaccine against the disease. These outbreaks indicated the need for a booster vaccine, which, as per its name, enhanced the first vaccine. It was administered between 12-19 years of age. The booster vaccine was still administered as MMR. The second dose reduced the reported cases of the disease even more. The country continued to fight against the disease. In 2000, America had successfully eliminated the disease. A country has to have had the continuous absence of the disease for 12 consecutive months to gain the state of the elimination of a disease. This means that no case and transmission occur within the nation. However, there can be infections from other countries. Let us not forget that the disease was still affecting people in most parts of the world, especially in the developing world. There were insufficient vaccines in emerging countries, which made the unvaccinated susceptible to the infection. Between 2001 and 2003, 216 new measles cases were recorded in the USA. Of all these cases, 96 were imported from other countries, while the others were indigenous. America reported 16 cases between 2001 and 2003. Was the disease becoming a nightmare again? These events show how difficult it may be to eliminate a viral infection from a country because it may still be contracted from other countries. Furthermore, the existing strains of the virus in the country may undergo mutation, causing outbreaks. In 2016, the World Health Organization reported an alarming increase in the number of people infected with measles. The world was witnessing what seemed to be the comeback of measles, which was once a global threat. In 2018, the world recorded a 300% rise in the number of cases of this disease. The most affected countries included Madagascar, the Philippines, Yemen, and Brazil. In 2019, things got worse, and although other global events may have shadowed it, the disease was afflicting many people. Take, for instance, Madagascar; it had 69,000 measles cases and 1,200 measles-related deaths. The Philippines witnessed 19,000 incidents, while Ukraine had to deal with a staggering 72,000 cases. One may wonder why this disease is taking such a heavy toll on some parts of the world. Here are some of the reasons why; the first reason is vaccine-refusal. Many people in the world refuse to take vaccines, mostly due to their religious faith. For instance, some parents are against vaccination; they are commonly known as anti-vax parents. When their unvaccinated children get exposed to measles, they catch the virus and go down with measles. Jewish communities are also known for their refusal of vaccines. In January 2019, the community had 700 cases of measles in Rockland and New York City during the measles outbreak that happened in the USA. Many children were affected, and they ended up requiring intensive care. This is sad because vaccines are available, but people shun them in the name of faith. Conspiracy theories are common in our world, where information spreads with the speed of lightning. One of these theories state that vaccines cause autism; many people have taken up this theory to be true. The theorists have been successful in convincing people not to vaccinate their children. Nevertheless, their success is also their setback because the unvaccinated children and adults are usually the ones hit hardest when outbreaks occur. In fact, most of them become so contagious and affect many people. Some people are hesitant to take the vaccine against measles. This complacency is mainly witnessed in younger parents who never had to witness the horrific face of this disease. They were born when the vaccine was already in use. Some have never even seen a patient suffering from measles, let alone the death caused by the malady. With such naivety, it is hard to convince them to vaccinate their children. They assume that fewer cases of the disease mean less threat. As they said, a little knowledge is dangerous. All these factors are a significant setback in the fight against measles. By the end of 2019, several countries had lost state of measles elimination. These countries include the United Kingdom, Czech Republic, Greece, and Albania. Unless these notions are corrected, we will live to witness more cases of measles despite having the solution right in our hands. There is no specific treatment for measles. This fact should make people wary of the disease. The physicians work towards relieving the symptoms and giving the patient supportive care. The doctor may prescribe medication to do away with fever. The most common drug for this is ibuprofen. The doctor often recommends it to boost one's immunity to fight the virus. Plenty of fluids, especially oral rehydration salts (ORS), are administered to rehydrate the body. Vitamin A supplements are also given to rejuvenate the immune system. If the patient is coughing, a humidifier is prescribed to ease the cough and sore throat. All this is done in an attempt to strengthen the body so that it can fight the virus. If it succeeds in doing so, the patient recovers, and most of them never go down with measles again. If not, the patient may eventually succumb to the illness immediately or develop complications that are degenerative and eventually cause death. Some patients may realize that they have been exposed to measles and report to health personnel even before the presentation of any symptoms of the disease. Such cases are treated in two ways. First, the physician may administer a measles vaccine within 72 hours of exposure. The second option is administering a dose of immunoglobulins within six days of exposure. These proteins fight against the virus. It is essential to understand that measles may manifest in various ways, bringing forth the different types of measles. Common measles is the disease that we described earlier in this text. Atypical measles occurs when someone who had been earlier inoculated using a killed virus develops measles after exposure to the disease. It was common in the 1960s. It occurs due to the failure of the body to develop immunity against measles. Modified measles arises when someone who has been administered with immunoglobulins after exposure to measles develops the disease. It also applies to children who come down with the disease despite still having some passive immunity from the immunoglobulins received from the mother. Modified measles is usually milder than typical measles. Hemorrhagic measles is a rare type of measles which is generally very severe. It causes high fever, seizures, and as the name suggests, bleeding into the mucous membranes and the skin. Prevention is definitely better than cure. How can we protect ourselves from contracting this disease, which seems to be getting ready for a hell of a comeback? The best and surest way to steer clear of the disease is by getting vaccinated against the disease. Herd immunity is best achieved by vaccination. This practice is done by ensuring that at least 90% of the population is vaccinated against measles. This way, there are incredibly low chances that anyone will get infected with the disease. Consequently, the rate of transmission is also minimal. It is, therefore, the task of the members of the community to urge everyone to be vaccinated and to get the booster vaccine. However, the measles vaccine should never be administered to immuno-compromised people, including pregnant women, PLWHA, people undergoing cancer treatment, or those that are taking medication that suppresses the immunity such as steroids. The virus is a live-attenuated virus that can actually become strong and attack their bodies in their state. This precaution applies to people who have had violent, life-threatening reactions to components of the vaccine or the vaccine as a whole. There are other methods that one can use to avoid measles. Good hand hygiene is one of these methods whereby one should wash their hands after visiting the toilet and before eating. People should avoid sharing their personal items with people suspected of being ill. This includes combs, toothbrushes, and eating utensils. They should also avoid direct contact with the ailing patient. These ways will minimize the risk of contracting the disease. If one realizes that they may be suffering from measles, the first step is always to seek immediate medical attention. They should not panic because the disease is manageable with the right care and support. Furthermore, the patients should avoid direct contact with other people to prevent transmitting the virus to them. They should work or study from home and avoid all public places until they are proven to be no longer contagious. They should cover their nose while coughing or sneezing to avoid releasing droplets containing the virus to the air. They should avoid being close to immuno-compromised people so that they may not transmit the disease to them. Measles is a disease that the human race has fought and stamped beneath their feet earlier. We should urge all to take the necessary precaution to avoid its resurgence, which means more suffering. May we not fight a fight that is unnecessary just because some people think that the opponent was unworthy or never existed at all. There are more diseases to be challenged, some of which the vaccines have not yet been developed, let alone the cure. Let us, therefore, make use of the available resources and eliminate measles from our various countries. Step by step, we may eventually eradicate measles from the globe, as hard as it may seem.

Dengue Fever

Dengue Fever is a disease that has been with human beings for ages. The condition was first mentioned in Chinese documents in 992 AD. The physicians described it as a water disease because the disease mostly affected those who dwelled near water sources. It was also present in Indian civilization as early as in the 18th century. In the 1780s, there were outbreaks of this disease that co-occurred in Africa, Asia, and Europe. In 1789, a physician, Benjamin Rush, coined the term 'break-bone fever' due to its symptoms of myalgia and arthralgia. Myalgia is a pain in several muscles at the same time, which is a characteristic of this disease. Arthralgia is a pain in the joints. The term Dengue is Spanish in origin. The Swahili people of East Africa coined the name 'Ka-Dinga pepo' from the word Dengue. The term Dengue means fastidious or careful. Such was the behavior of the sufferers of this disease, which was caused by bone and muscle pain. The disease also afflicted slaves in the West Indies. They called it Dandy Fever because the disease caused one to have the gait and posture of a dandy. In as much as the disease continuously afflicted the human race, the relationship between the disease and mosquito as the vector was only established as late as in the 20th century. Today, we understand that the pathogen, Dengue virus is transmitted to humans through a bite. The vectors are primarily the mosquitoes of the species *Aedes aegypti*. Dengue Fever virus DENV is a flavivirus of the genus *Flaviviridae*. The virus is enveloped and contains genetic material in the form of single-stranded positive-sense RNA. The virus is in the same family as the White Nile Virus, Yellow Fever virus, Tick-Borne Encephalitis virus, among others. The virus exists as four different types known as serotypes. These types are differentiated from each other by the use of surface proteins. They are; DENV-1, DENV-2, DENV-3, and DENV-4. The viruses have 50-70% homology and cause almost the same symptoms; Dengue Fever, Dengue Hemorrhagic, and Dengue Shock Syndrome. The symptoms of the disease range from acute and manageable to severe and life-threatening. Dengue Fever is a disease that is known to have afflicted military personnel, especially in tropical countries, as well as the inhabitants of these countries. Let us focus on the US military. In 1898, during the Spanish-American War, the US military was stationed in several countries, including Cuba, Puerto Rico, Panama, and the Philippines. In these countries, many sorts of new maladies were afflicting the military personnel. The diseases included Typhoid, Yellow Fever, and Malaria. In these countries, the mosquitoes of the species *Aedes aegypti* were common. They were the vectors of most of the diseases that afflicted the army. The military did not see Dengue Fever as a priority because the illness had a low mortality rate. The disease was also misdiagnosed as other febrile diseases several times. All doubts concerning the viciousness of the disease were dissolved in 1897 when a Dengue Fever epidemic erupted in Cuba. In as much as the mortality rate was low, many soldiers were weak, and this undermined their position in the conquest. In the following three years, Dengue Fever outbreaks occurred severally in Texas and Florida in the USA. These events highlighted the effects that the disease could have on a population. In the Philippines, the Army Tropical Diseases Board was created to investigate the health issues which were affecting the US army as well as the local inhabitants. Initially, Dengue Fever was not a priority for them. They said that it caused a low, constant non-effective rate among the troops and was not a cause for alarm. However, in 1906, a Dengue Fever epidemic occurred at Fort William McKinley in Manila, and it hugely enervated the military. This incident showed the military the gravity of the threat that the disease posed. Consequently, the Army Tropical Disease Board took a keen interest in studying the disease. The Philippines tour of duty, which occurred every two years, played a significant role in understanding Dengue Fever's occurrence. The board realized that hospitalizations for Dengue Fever were about 101 per 1000 persons. When the new troops arrived, 40% of the soldiers contracted the disease within a year. The disease recurred within one year for 30% of the soldiers and 15% of those staying for more than two years, and the illness recurred a third time. They also realized that the infection occurred mostly in Manila and the surrounding urban environment. It was less common in the camps located in remote places. During the Second World War, Dengue Fever was the second most threatening tropical disease after malaria. Epidemics were breaking out in several parts of the world, especially those with a tropical climate. It profoundly affected military activities. This was mainly because it afflicted many soldiers at the same time and weakened them for about three weeks. It made the army incur extra costs, especially in the evacuation of military personnel who had been affected by the disease. Word of Dengue Fever spread far and wide, especially to the troops that were in the tropical areas. In 1943, in Hawaii, the disease was reintroduced after 30 years of absence by commercial airplanes from Honolulu. The disease was first reported in the Waikiki area. This outbreak prompted the US military to take immediate action because they knew far too well the effects such a virus could have on their position in battle. First, the area was declared as off-limits to the troops. Local authorities inspected people's homes from door to door to understand the gravity of the situation. They also provided health education on how to prevent Dengue Fever. Mosquito control was enhanced in the area, and this practice extended to other parts of Hawaii, including the cities and towns. More areas were identified as having the disease, and the troops were prohibited from visiting such areas. These incidents show the impact that a disease can have on the military, and consequently, the political position of a country. After the Second World War, the world witnessed more Dengue Fever outbreaks than ever before. It was attributed to the enormous urbanization that was taking place. The towns were often not well planned, and this promoted stagnant of water, which provided breeding grounds for *Aedes aegypti*, the vector of the disease. Many people suffered from the disease, and this prompted more measures to curb the spread of the disease as well as manage the existing cases. The other factors that increased the spread of the disease could have been climate change, poor mosquito control, and increased international travel. Let us look at how the Dengue Fever virus is transmitted from a sick person to a healthy one considering that the disease is non-communicable. The transmission occurs when a mosquito bites an ill person. As it sucks blood, it takes the virus from the infected person because the virus circulates in the bloodstream. The virus remains within the body of the mosquito for as long as the mosquito continues living. When the mosquito lands on a healthy person, it releases the virus via its saliva as it sucks blood. This way, the virus enters the bloodstream of a healthy person. It does this to every Dengue Fever free person it encounters within its short life. Mosquitoes can spread the virus so fast, and they are the reason why epidemics occur. The *Aedes aegypti* is a very dangerous mosquito species because, unlike other mosquitoes, it feeds during the daytime when people's activities are at the peak. The female feeds multiple times a day in the egg-laying period, and what's more astonishing is that once it lays eggs, they can remain viable for a couple of months. Despite the environment that they are in, they always hatch when they come in contact with water. This way, the species continue surviving despite the harshest environments. Unfortunately, *Aedes aegypti* is not the only mosquito species that we should be wary of. *Aedes albopictus* is a secondary vector of the Dengue Fever virus. Initially, it was mainly found in Asia but has now spread to Europe and America and a small part of Africa thanks to the trade of items such as used tires and lucky bamboo. This strain is equally dangerous due to its ability to adapt to different climates and efficiently spread the disease. This species feeds on a wide variety of hosts; therefore, it can bridge zoonotic pathogens and introduce them to humans. Apart from the Dengue Fever virus, it is also a vector to the Chikungunya virus and Dirofilaria. There is also a possibility that the disease could be transmitted from mother to child during pregnancy. In as much as vertical transmission rarely occurs, when it does, its effects may be lethal to the unborn baby. It may cause preterm labor, low weight at birth, or even fetal distress. This is the reason why pregnant mothers are advised to avoid this disease at all costs. At times, Dengue Fever may not directly affect the fetus but cause deterioration in the mother's health, which affects the fetus' health and may end the fetus's life. Once one is affected by Dengue Fever, they undergo an incubation period of about 4-10 days. After this period, they can develop either of the two types of Dengue Fever; Dengue Fever with or without symptoms, or severe Dengue Fever. The symptoms of Dengue Fever last about 2-7 days. The symptoms are initially flu-like, and this may cause one to underestimate the danger posed by this disease. Dengue Fever should be suspected when someone develops a high fever of about 40 degrees Celsius. During this febrile phase, there are a couple of other symptoms that occur. These symptoms are: severe headache, pain behind the eyes, muscle and joint pain, and nausea. These signs may wrongly indicate the flu, and many people recover at this phase even if they are untreated. When such cases occur, there are fewer numbers of reported Dengue Fever cases, and this leads to an underestimation of the burden of the disease in the community. Moreover, such patients and asymptomatic patients can also contribute to the spread of the disease unknowingly when bitten by mosquitoes. The second phase of Dengue Fever is a critical phase which occurs 3-7 days after the onset of the illness. The fever is dropping to about 38 degrees Celsius, giving the patient a false sense of hope. At this stage, most patients develop warning signs of the disease, which can advance to fatal complications. The patient has severe abdominal pain and persistent vomiting, which makes it difficult for the patient to take food or medication. The patient breathes rapidly. They have bleeding gums; their vomit contains blood too. The patient develops fatigue but becomes restless. At this stage, the patient should seek immediate medical care without which the patient develops a fatal complication. These complications include: plasma leaking, fluid accumulation in the lungs leading to respiratory distress, severe bleeding, or organ impairment. Once one has contracted and fought off a particular serotype of the Dengue virus, the body develops antibodies against it. Remember that all the four serotypes have 50-70% homology in their structure. Therefore, when the same serotype attacks the body, it can efficiently fight off the virus using the antibodies. It can also produce more of these particular antibodies, which eventually overwhelms the virus. However, if another serotype attacks, the antibodies act up against the body. The new serotypes homology with the previous one tricks the body. The body produces and releases the antibodies that fought off the last serotype successfully. Nonetheless, these antibodies do not affect the new serotype, and it attacks the body severely. This phenomenon explains why the disease continues to cause suffering even in endemic communities. Just like the majority of viral diseases, Dengue Fever has no specific treatment. The physicians provide medication to relieve the symptoms of the illness. These drugs, coupled with proper supportive care, lead to the recovery of the body from the disease. Fever relievers are used to calm the febrile reaction that the body exhibits during Dengue infections. Pain killers are used in relieving muscle and body aches as well as abdominal pains. The recommended pain relievers are paracetamol or acetaminophen, while non-steroidal anti-inflammatory drugs (NSAIDs) such as ibuprofen should be avoided. The NSAIDs work by thinning the blood, and this may trigger hemorrhage or worsen existing bleeding making the disease very hard to manage. All in all, maintenance of the healthy levels of bodily fluids is critical, especially in patients with Hemorrhagic Dengue Fever. To ensure that the patients recover quickly with minimal disruption of bodily functions, patients should seek medical care in the early phases of the sickness. Dengue Fever reported cases have increased 15-fold over the last 20 years. For a disease that is more often than not mistaken for other febrile diseases or is asymptomatic, it is accurate to say that the cases may be much more than the number. Today, 3.9 billion people are at the risk of Dengue Fever infection around the world. The WHO estimates that 390 million infections occur per year, whether symptomatic or asymptomatic, reported or not. Of these infections, 96 million are manifested clinically and are often the only reported cases. The disease mostly affects Asia, even though 129 countries are at risk of infection. The disease is a cause for alarm; before 1970, only nine countries had been afflicted by the disease; today, 100 countries are endemic to the disease. The nations are distributed throughout Africa, the Middle East, Asia, Europe, and America. It is necessary, therefore, that every global citizen gain access to information about the disease, and most importantly, knows how to control its spread. The year 2019 saw the largest number of cases globally. Some countries, such as Afghanistan, recorded cases of the disease for the first time in history. In the American region, 3.1 million cases were reported, 25,000 of which were classified as severe Dengue. However, unlike the previous years, the deaths associated with this malady dramatically decreased. Prevention of Dengue Fever is critical in both virgin and endemic populations. The primary method of prevention is the control of mosquitoes. If mosquito bites can be avoided, transmission from the infected persons to Dengue Free people can be effectively stalled. This would mean that only existing Dengue Fever cases would be requiring medical attention. The most significant step in controlling mosquitoes is by controlling their breeding. This measure can be achieved by denying them access to their breeding places. We can accomplish this by ensuring there is no stagnant water in the environment. Domestic water storage containers should be emptied and cleaned weekly to that effect. They should also be covered always. We should dispose of solid waste properly as well as remove man-made artificial habitats that can hold water. Appropriate insecticides can be sprayed to outdoor water containers to ensure the elimination of the mosquitoes that may shelter there. By preventing the mosquitoes from breeding, we can be sure to deal with only one generation of mosquitoes, and this plays a significant role in the control of this disease. The mosquito, *Aedes aegypti*, is known for attacking and biting during the day. It attacks the majority of people when they are up and about. In the bustle of the day, one only realizes the damage after the mosquito has already had its fair share of blood. At home, work, or school, specific measures should be put in place to protect individuals from mosquitoes. Mosquito coils, vaporizers, and repellent creams should be used to drive away mosquitoes. Window screens should be put in place to prevent the insects from entering buildings. Everyone should wear clothes that minimize exposure to mosquitoes, especially if they are not wearing repellent creams. The community should be knowledgeable about Dengue Fever and all that pertains to it. When the community has the needed information, the people can efficiently protect themselves from the virus. Knowledge is the most potent weapon required to fight any disease. There is a new flame of hope because the vaccine for the Dengue virus is now in use. Dengvaxia, which was invented in 2019, is now available in many parts of the world. The vaccine is a live attenuated virus and has been licensed for administration to persons between the age of 9 and 45 years in several countries. Unlike other vaccines, WHO and the developer, Sanofi Pasteur, recommend the administration of the vaccine to people who have already suffered from the disease, at least once. Unlike vaccines for most infections, if Dengvaxia is used by people who have not contracted the disease before, they may develop severe Dengue if they get infected by the virus later naturally. The virus, therefore, protects those who have already contracted the disease from contracting it another time. For full effect, three doses of the vaccine are taken six months apart. The vaccine comes in handy because the number of endemic countries is on a steady rise, but with the immunization, the disease may be effectively contained. The governments of endemic countries have received immense support from the World Health Organization while dealing with Dengue Fever. Both endemic and new countries have witnessed the organization at play, especially in the prevention, control, and treatment of Dengue Fever. The WHO provides technical support and guidance in the management of outbreaks of Dengue Fever. It supports countries to improve their health and reporting system to know the actual burden of the disease and bear it sufficiently. The organization also collects the official reports of the cases of the disease in all the member countries. It then publishes guidelines on how to handle cases of the disease, how to diagnose, prevent and control it, and makes them available to all the member states—the WHO has contributed enormously to the management of Dengue Fever. As citizens of the world, we have made significant progress in the management of Dengue Fever. Since the number of those at risk of contracting the disease grows daily, we have the necessary information on how to stay safe or get treated. Moreover, we have a vaccine, which is very crucial in preventing the reoccurrence of the malady. All we need to do is; take the necessary precautions, stay in a healthy environment, and most importantly, be informed. We can eradicate this disease!

HIV/AIDS

HIV originated in Kinshasa, Congo, in the 1920s when it crossed species from chimpanzees to human beings. The people hunted these animals, and they could have contracted the disease by coming into contact with the chimpanzees' blood. Before the 1980s, the number of people that contracted the disease remains unknown. It was in the 1980s when the disease was in the limelight for causing such despondency to mankind. From then up to now, there is no cure for this illness. HIV/AIDS continues to be a pandemic that scars people for life, making sure to follow them up to the grave. You have probably heard of HIV, but what is this virus that continues to wreak havoc in the four corners of the globe? HIV stands for Human Immunodeficiency Virus. It is a virus, specifically a retrovirus. The virus contains genetic material known as RNA contained in an envelope. RNA, which stands for ribonucleic acid, is a five-carbon sugar-acid contained in HIV's genetic make-up. When HIV infects the body, it attacks the immune system leading to a syndrome called Acquired Immune Deficiency Syndrome (AIDS). In 1981, in America, some homosexuals were diagnosed with Pneumocystis Pneumonia. The disease was caused by Pneumocystis Jiroveci, a harmless fungus found in the body. This infection indicated that the patients were immuno-suppressed. By the following year, The New York Times reported that the disorder had affected 335 people and killed 136 of them. The CDC named it gay-related immune deficiency or GRID. Others called it the gay plague. Homosexuals faced immense discrimination and prejudice in general. Little did the people know that the disease could affect anyone of any gender, age, or color. Some men in New York and California were diagnosed with Kaposi's sarcoma. In September 1982, the CDC coined the term AIDS. Later in the year, several European countries reported cases of AIDS. The New York Times published about the people at high risk of contracting the illness were nick-named 'The Four-H club.' It comprised hemophiliacs, homosexuals, heroin users, and people of Haitian origin.

Hemophiliacs are people whose blood doesn't clot normally and therefore lose too much blood because of an injury. They need blood transfusions to maintain healthy levels. Most of them had received HIV-infected blood unknowingly, and they had AIDS. Homosexuals were the first to be diagnosed with the disease. As time went by, more and more gay men were diagnosed with the sickness making them a risk population. Heroin users were identified as a risk population because most of them shared infected needles to administer the drug. Moreover, scientists later discovered that when the users were drugged, most of them would engage in irresponsible sexual activities risking contraction of the disease. By the time the media was publicizing the Four-H idea, most of the people living with HIV/AIDS were Haitians. This situation made most people think that they were at a higher risk of contracting the illness. However, it was later established that the disease could infect one and all, indiscriminately. When one contracts the illness, they develop flu-like symptoms. These are fever, headache, chills, sore throat, swollen lymph nodes, and fatigue. At this stage, the disease is defined as Acute Retroviral Syndrome. From there, the condition becomes asymptomatic until it develops to AIDS. At this stage, the flu-like symptoms have already disappeared. The immune system cannot eliminate HIV and therefore tolerates it. At this stage, many people are not yet aware that they have the infection. HIV destroys white blood cells, particularly the CD4 cells. CD4 cells are white blood cells whose cell surface marker is CD4. The destruction of CD4 cells weakens the immune system drastically. The lower the CD4 count, the more the chances of attack by opportunistic infections. Opportunistic infections are not harmful in a person with a competent immune system. However, their attack may be fatal to immuno-suppressed individuals. When the CD4 count is low, and the viral load is high, many people develop complications such as Pulmonary pneumonia, TB, cervical cancer, among others. At this stage, the disease is chronic, and the patient has to strive to manage the disease and lead what they deem to be a normal life. The pestilence may render one bed-ridden and cause their body to waste; thus, they become unable to work. Other than afflicting physical pain, the disease may indirectly cause mental problems. The patients often suffer stigma from people in society. From the workspace, schools, homes, and religious places, people living with HIV/AIDS (PLWHA) are treated differently, and at times, unfairly. This lowers their self-esteem, and the majority wish for death. However, with endless love, support, and encouragement, the people can overcome and live a better life. The number of people infected with the disease grew daily. Some countries in Asia reported several cases of the disease. In Africa, previously unaffected countries started reporting incidences of the disease. Doctors in Uganda described it as a fatal wasting condition that the local people called 'slim.' By the end of the year, many people, aware of the danger they were facing, set up several AIDS-specific organizations. San Francisco AIDS Foundation (SFAF) and Terrence Higgins Trust are examples of such organizations. In January 1983, contrary to what the people had initially believed, female partners of men living with AIDS were reported to be having the disease. This discovery confirmed the fear that the virus could be transmitted via heterosexual sex. Doctors who had been studying the disease at Pasteur Institute in France discovered some astonishing facts about the virus. First, they established that it was a retrovirus, which means that its genetic material consists of RNA. The virus, therefore, used the body-cells' machinery to construct DNA from RNA, then, multiply and invade more body cells. They also named it Lymphadenopathy-Associated Virus (LAV). They suggested that this virus could be the cause of AIDS. In June of the same year, some children were diagnosed with AIDS, implying that the disease could be passed on via casual contact. WHO ruled out these claims and established that most of the children contracted it during pregnancy from the mothers, while suckling, during labor or shortly after. By

September 1983, the CDC (Center for Disease Control and Prevention) established the methods of transmission of the disease. This includes; sexual intercourse, blood transfusion, and sharing of sharp objects such as non-sterile dental objects. Some routes of transmission, such as food, water, air, and casual contact, were ruled out by the CDC. The CDC, in an attempt to protect health care workers and other allied health professionals, published and publicized the first set of recommended precautions for the prevention of AIDS transmission. Towards the end of the year, AIDS was recognized as a global pandemic. In November, WHO met for the first time to access the global AIDS situation and began surveillance. For instance, they realized that by the end of 1983, 3,064 Americans had HIV, and 1,292 of them died. Many institutions around the globe continued to research about HIV/AIDS. Each day the institutions discovered something new, they shed more light. In April 1984, the world took a significant step relating to the AIDS pandemic. The National Cancer Institute announced that HTLV-III, a retrovirus, was the cause of AIDS. They then had a joint conference with the Pasteur Institute in France, whereby they declared that HTLV-III and LAV were genetically similar and were the cause of AIDS. A blood test known as the ELISA to screen was widely used for the virus. By that time, scientists were hoping for the development of the vaccine within two years. In 1985, the Food and Drugs Association (FDA) approved it. Numerous HIV tests have been developed. The tests use blood, urine, or saliva. They all detect HIV antibodies to confirm the presence of the virus; however, blood tests are usually faster due to the high amounts of antibodies. AIDS caused a high death toll. In 1985, Rock Hudson was the first celebrity to die from the disease. This incident, in conjunction with the death of many other people, caused terror to reign supreme. For instance, people in the USA had the fear that HIV would make its way to the blood banks, and this would cause the infection of many people. The FDA, therefore, banned gay men from donating blood, and this regulation went on for 30 years until 2015, where they were allowed to do so. However, they have to have been celibate for a whole year. Blood banks were also screened regularly to avoid infection to the receptors. The monstrosity spread far and wide with the speed of a bush fire. By the end of 1985, each nation had at least a case of AIDS, bringing the total to 20,000 people. The mid-1980s is the period with the peak numbers of people living with HIV/AIDS. This could be because people didn't have enough knowledge concerning the illness, its mode of transmission, and its effect. In some cases, those who got the information assumed that it was propaganda, ignored all precautions, and for these mistakes, they paid dearly. Scientists developed the first antiretroviral medication for HIV. It was called azidothymidine (AZT). Since then, much progress has happened, and different types of Antiretrovirals (ARV) have been manufactured. Examples of ARVs include Nucleoside reverse transcriptase inhibitor (NRTIs). These work by inhibiting the conversion of RNA to DNA in the virus. These drugs stall the reproduction of the virus, therefore reducing its virulence. Zidovudine, Tenofovir disoproxil, and Lamivudine are examples of NRTIs. Non-nucleoside based reverse transcriptase inhibitors (NNRTIs) are another type of ARVs. The inhibit transcriptase activity by binding to it directly and blocking the process of transcription. Reverse Transcriptase is the enzyme that catalyzes the conversion or transcription of RNA to DNA. NNRTIs include; Doravine, Efavirenz, Etravine, and Rilpivirine. Integrase inhibitors are a group of ARVs that target an enzyme called integrase. Integrase is essential for viral replication. Inhibiting viral replication slows down its propagation and spread in the body. Examples of integrase inhibitors include; Raltegravir, Elvitegravir, and Dolutegravir. Another type of ARVs is Entry inhibitors, which stop HIV from entering the cell. They occur in two forms; CCR5 inhibitors and fusion inhibitors. For the virus to enter the cell, it has to bind two receptors on the cell surface, the CD4 and CCR5 receptors. CCR5 inhibitors bind the CCR5 receptors, blocking HIV from accessing the cell. Fusion inhibitors block fusion in as much as the virus may have attached CD4 and CCR5 receptors. The Entry inhibitors deny HIV access to the cell. The virus, therefore, cannot use the cell's machinery to replicate and spread to other parts of the body. There are different types of ARVs, and they are the single-tablet regimen, booster drugs, and protease inhibitors. ARVs have played a significant role in ensuring that the people living with HIV/AIDS live a quality and fulfilling life. In recent years, they have become readily available in many parts of the world. The World Health Organization estimated that 400,000 people were living with HIV/AIDS in 1988, and 100,000 of them were living in the USA. WHO also declared December 1, as World AIDS Day. The 1990s was a period of creation of vast awareness of the disease among the people. In 1991, Marc Happel, a costume designer, invented the red ribbon as the symbol for AIDS, and this symbol reminds people of the presence of the disease in the globe. In this period, people still had the misconception that AIDS was a gay person's' disease. Freddie Mercury, a lead singer in the band Queen, tried to dispel it by declaring that he had the disease. Unfortunately, he passed away the following day. In 1993, the USA banned HIV-infected persons from entering the country. In this year, cervical cancer, pulmonary tuberculosis, and recurrent tuberculosis were added to the list of HIV indicators. WHO estimated 700,000 people with HIV in the Pacific and Asia. There were 2.5 million cases globally. The year 1994 was a time of breakthrough in the prevention of mother-child HIV transmission. AZT was approved for this use. This medication prevented very many unborn and newborn children from contracting the disease. In December, the FDA approved the use of the oral-HIV test. This test was the first non-blood HIV test. The following year the FDA mandated the use of the first protease inhibitors. These were the early Highly Active Antiretroviral Therapy (HAART).

Today, HAART is the fundamental component in the care of PLWHA. HAART has proven to be effective in that it immediately caused the decline of deaths of HIV/AIDS to 60%-80%. There were 4.7 million new HIV infections around the globe by the end of 1995. Of these new infections, 2.5 million occurred in Asia and 1.9 in Africa. The year 1996 was a time of more optimism despite the rising cases of HIV/AIDS. 23 million people around the globe were living with AIDS. The world was making enormous progress in the management of HIV/AIDS. HAART was reported to be effective in the 11th International AIDS Conference held in Vancouver. In as much as the cure was not yet found, the people on treatment regimens led a healthy, better life. This year also ushered the first home testing kit for the viral load of HIV in the blood. This was helpful since patients could detect the deterioration of health even before the manifestation of the effects. The first NNRTI known as nevirapine gained approval by the FDA that year. It was during this year that the FDA approved the first HIV urine test. Eastern Europe, China, and Cambodia reported new HIV infections. In 1997, significant advancement was seen in Antiretroviral therapy. FDA sanctioned Combivir for use by PLWHA. Combivir is a combination of two ARV tablets that are taken each day as a single tablet. This tablet makes the taking of medicine less tedious. There were about 16,000 new infections daily, which lead to a total of 30 million PLWHA at the end of the year. By the end of 1999, 33 million people were living with this malady, and this was quite alarming. The WHO declared it as the fourth most prominent cause of death in the world. In as much as the ARV therapy was effective in suppressing the disease, it was quite expensive. In developing countries, only the very fortunate could afford it. Therefore, the disease continued to wreak havoc in all corners of the globe, especially in developing countries. In 2000, pharmaceutical companies were urged by UNAIDS to waiver the price for the developing countries. More people now had access to the

ARVs, and this significantly reduced the death toll in these countries. Since it was a new millennium, the United Nations had an elaborate plan in improving healthcare in the world. In September 2000, the UN declared the Millennium Development Goals, which included; reversing the spread of HIV, malaria, which affected almost all countries in the tropical regions and TB. The combat against HIV/AIDS was strenuous, and it drained the majority of the developing countries financially. In 2001, the UN General Assembly suggested the creation of a 'Global Fund.' The fund was to help the nations to combat the pandemic while maintaining financial stability. WHO allowed countries to manufacture their own generic ARVs. ARVs became more affordable and accessible, and since then, the combat against HIV has become more manageable. In the 2000s, the testing of the disease has become more efficient and effective, thanks to the rapid HIV tests that are available. The year 2005 saw the highest number of deaths due to AIDS, with more than 3 million globally. There was also a vast number of people living with the disease, 40 million people. The situation was utterly devastating, for the governments and individuals alike. In 2006, male circumcision proved to lower the chances of male to female HIV transmission by 60%. In the 2010s, there was the development of pre and post-exposure anaphylaxis. These are regimens that reduce the risk of one getting contracting HIV after exposure. They prevent the virus from establishing itself in the body. In this era, it was also found out that the starting of the ARV treatment early reduced transmission by 96%. In 2011, Complera was approved for use, increasing the variety for the PLWHA. In 2014, UNAIDS aimed to eliminate AIDS as a pandemic. They sought to do this using the Fast Track Strategy, whereby they would increase HIV treatment and Prevention programs drastically. They aim to achieve the following; diagnose 90% of PLWHA, 90% of the diagnosed people to access ART (antiretroviral therapy), and 90% of those accessing ART to achieve viral suppression. The fight against

HIV/AIDS yielded fruits. In 2015, the Millennium Development Goal concerning HIV/AIDS was overwhelmingly achieved six months before the due date. The halting and the reversal of the spread of HIV had been achieved. WHO released new treatment guidelines whereby all patients who test positive for HIV should start ART immediately after diagnosis regardless of their CD4 count. In October, UNAIDS released the new global goal concerning HIV/AIDS management. This was known as Sustainable Development Goals. UNAIDS called for improvement and speeding up of the global HIV response to achieve HIV prevention and treatment targets. The nations were to strive to achieve zero discrimination. We may not have discovered a cure for AIDS, but the progress that has been made in the management of the malady is remarkable. The development is due to the hard work of scientists, the relentlessness of health care workers, and the commitment of the patients. The governments have also given undying support to the organizations mentioned above. The WHO, the organizations that are part of it, and other regional organizations have contributed immensely to this progress through financial support and follow up. With the current pace, the set goals will be achieved in a huge way. Some people live with HIV, but all of us are affected and at risk of contracting the disease. We should all unite our efforts in fighting this disease. Our unity decides whether it is here to stay or just a passing cloud.

Schistosomiasis

Schistosomiasis is a parasitic disease with both acute and chronic clinical presentations. It is also called bilharzia or bilharziasis. It is caused by trematode worms or blood flukes of the genus *Schistosoma*. There are various species implicated in the causation of this condition, and they are *S. haematobium, S. japonicum, and S. mansoni*, among many other documented species. The last two are majorly causative in the intestinal and hepatic forms of the disease, whereas haematobium is implicated in urogenital schistosomiasis. It is important to note that this is a disease that has evolved with humans over a long period. Ancient writings in the Egyptian medical papyri describe disease presentation that depicts the clinical presentation of bilharziasis. Moreover, among other ancient documents, the Assyrian medical records give symptoms that point to the same condition. This dates back to around 1500 B.C. In the Bible, there are reported cases of the same disease that the residents of the then Mesopotamia termed to be a punishment or a condition that affected a person who was cursed. Various archaeological shreds of evidence have tried to confirm the same old-age disease, such as the dating back of schistosome remains in mummies in Egypt. Therefore, this depicts a parasitic infection that has haunted humans for ages, especially those living in or near swampy areas, near water basins, or in wetlands. The implicated causative agent, as stated earlier, are the trematode worms or blood flukes. These parasites have two hosts that help them to complete their life cycles. These are the intermediate and definitive hosts. The snails are the definitive hosts, and humans act as the definitive hosts. Other primates and apes are also thought to act as the definitive hosts. The schistosomes are thought to survive up to 40 years in a definitive host. During its life cycle, the schistosomes move from their habitats in water-based grounds into the snails and finally mature and grow within the human body. Once mature within the human body, the male species mates with the female ones. Finally, the female lays eggs into the lining of intestines or bladder, which are eventually passed out with feces and urine to freshwater for the start of another life-cycle. People get infected during their daily activities that involve water. These are farming, swimming, fishing in infested water. Poor hygiene and playing practices, especially among children, predispose them to infection as they come in contact with water containing the intermediate hosts. By contact with the water, humans come in contact with the larval forms of schistosomes and are ingested into the human body. Within the body, these larvae develop into adult forms that live in the blood vessels where the females lay eggs. As stated earlier, some of the eggs are shed off from the body through urine and feces. The remaining eggs initiate an immune reaction in the body, which eventually causes organ damage. The organs damaged are mainly the liver, bladder, and the intestines. Schistosomiasis commonly occurs in the tropical and subtropical regions affecting people in rural communities. Those in areas with poor sanitation and poor hygiene conditions are likely to contract the disease. Lack of access to clean water leads to one contracting the disease, which is commonly seen among the poor communities, such as Africa. There are acute cases reported among tourists visiting this region. Children are more vulnerable to this disease due to their playful nature. Whereas for women, those participating in daily chores using water drawn from infested water points, there is an increased risk of contracting the disease and even HIV in cases of urogenital schistosomiasis. Of all the cases of schistosomiasis in the world, 90% of them requiring treatment occur in Africa. This shows that the prevalence of the disease is higher in this region. This is because a greater part of the population practice farming, fishing, or use water from rivers and lakes for domestic duties. Symptoms of bilharzia vary depending on the infested organs. For the intestinal and hepatic forms of schistosomiasis, the organs affected are mainly within the gastrointestinal tract. The mechanism of organ destruction remains the same for both forms of the disease. It is due to immune reactions to the eggs laid within the body. The patient presents with blood-stained stool, abdominal pains, and diarrhea. In advanced cases, there is an enlargement of the liver, commonly referred to as hepatomegaly. Due to this, there is perforation of peritoneal walls leading to an accumulation of fluid within the peritoneum. In later stages, a patient will present with increased blood pressure within the abdominal vessels, which eventually causes splenomegaly. A long-term complication will be the development of cancer of the liver. For the urogenital form of schistosomiasis, the classic symptom is blood in the urine. Hematuria is the commonest symptom that indicates the destruction of the urogenital tract. In advanced cases, there is fibrosis of the bladder, ureter, and kidney. For women, pain during sexual intercourse is a common complaint due to ulcers within the reproductive tract. In some cases, there is vaginal bleeding that could be spontaneous or occur during intercourse. For men, there is a destruction of the seminal vesicles and prostate glands, leading to decreased production of seminal fluid. The disease may also have a long-term complication of infertility. In 2000, WHO recorded an annual death rate of 200,000 patients globally. This indicates that, indeed, this is a serious condition with death as its possible outcome. However, the disease is notably a cause of disability than a killer. This condition impacts on the economy and socially on the affected community. For the affected children, the disease can cause pain and discomfort. Due to a characteristic loss of blood, the infants or pediatric patients could present with a complication of anemia. The discomfort impairs the child's ability to learn, cause stunted growth, and could even cause malnourishment. In chronic cases, a person's ability to do work is impaired due to chronic abdominal pains. This eventually impacts the person's productivity, which harms the local economy. Psychological torment due to bloodstains in human excreta can be tackled by proper advice, and with early treatment, such symptoms can cease. For most women, the pain during coitus can be uncomfortable and even affect the relationship with her partner of the opposite sex. A lowered self-esteem is common in females. The diagnosis of schistosomiasis begins with the taking of a good history of the patient and the presenting complaints. It is important to note the patient's residence, career, age, and common leisure activities. This helps in understanding whether they fall into the high-risk groups of contracting the disease. Moreover, the geographical location of the presenting patient is important to determine the likelihood of having the condition. The presenting complaint is then recorded, and the patient questioned further on any associated symptoms. A clinician can arrive at a provisional diagnosis just by using the clinical history. Definitive diagnosis is based on the detection of parasite eggs in feces and urine. These eggs are detected in the fecal matter through a technique that involves the use of methylene blue-stained cellophane soaked in glycerin or glass slides known as the Kato-Katz technique. For the detection of eggs in urine, a filtration technique is used. Using a nylon paper or polycarbonate filters is the standard method. For children with this condition, microscopic blood can be detected in urine using chemical reagent strips. For persons living in non-endemic areas, serological and immunological tests may be carried out to determine the exposure to infection and the need for thorough examination and follow-up. This is so important for tourists planning to visit or having a history of a visit to endemic areas. Large scale treatment of this disease is important in highly-endemic areas, which include about 50 countries identified by WHO. Praziquantel is the right drug for the treatment of bilharziasis. It is a broad-spectrum anthelmintic drug advocated for by WHO as a chemotherapeutic agent to treat active cases of the disease. It has rapid absorption in the gastrointestinal tract. It is metabolized in the liver and excreted through the urine and feces. Some of the documented benefits of praziquantel are its high efficacy, ease of administration, relative safety with mild to moderate side effects. Possible drug resistance has been observed with the use of this drug. This can be due to the inefficacy of the drug to treat the early stages of schistosomes with it. Poor compliance with the drug may also fail to achieve healing. Therefore, there has to be another alternative. This is common, especially with *S. mansoni*. The other alternative is oxamniquine, which has efficacy against the early stages of schistosomes and the *S. mansoni* strains. Just like praziquantel, oxamniquine has a relatively rapid absorption rate in the gut. As prevention is better than cure, all governments need to promote measures that will help prevent the occurrence of new cases of the disease. To avoid this disease, one has to avoid contact with water infested with the schistosomes species. This involves avoiding activities such as swimming or wading in pooled water following a rainy season or in water reservoirs. For communities that solely depend on the fetched water for domestic use, it's advisable to boil for more than a minute to kill the larvae. Other measures include filtering of water using a fine mesh. In cases where one cannot avoid contact with infested water, the application of insect repellants on the skin is advisable to prevent cutaneous penetration of the larvae. In areas with high endemicity, preventive chemotherapy should be administered. The at-risk groups to be given priority are the school going children, lactating, and pregnant women. Community awareness should be created in the endemic areas for the disease. This involves conducting educational campaigns on preventive measures to help evade the disease. Environmental hygiene is an important intervention in prevention. This is done through draining of any stagnant or pooled water, especially during the rainy season. For farmers working in swampy areas such as rice farms, they should put on protective wear such as gumboots to protect their skin from contacting the infective larval stages of schistosomes. Chemical spray of the water reservoirs can be done to kill the snails that act as intermediate hosts. The government can intervene by providing clean, piped water to the affected communities for domestic use. Another way is by constructing community-owned water cleaning plants to provide pure water for drinking. Currently, there are some WHO recommendations in response to schistosomiasis. This is an integrated approach that will help in curbing the disease in the areas within the tropics where the disease has a higher occurrence. First, preventive chemotherapy is advocated as a priority in its prevention. To co-ordinate this preventive strategy, partnership with other agencies such as research bodies, non-governmental organizations, governments of the affected countries, and the United Nations (UN) is paramount. This will help ease the enactment of the given policies. However, this body remains with the duty of developing technical guidelines and tools for use by national control programs. The drug of choice for preventive chemotherapy being praziquantel, its presence in the market for use, is important. World Health Organization has advocated for the production of an adequate amount of this drug. Annually, there are about 100 million orders made for this drug, as documented by WHO. One major problem encountered with this preventive chemotherapy is the inability to manage cases of re-infection. In conclusion, schistosomiasis is a parasitic disease common in the tropics, among the many tropical diseases burdening continents such as Africa and Asia, with Africa being greatly affected. With man being the definitive host of the pathogenic schistosomes, the concern of many is the potential of eventual disability on the infected person rather than the mortality of the disease. Schistosomiasis, being a water-borne disease, can be easily prevented by the avoidances of schistosomes infested water. Over the past 50 years, several measures have been put in place to curb the menace of bilharzia. World Health Organization advocates mainly for preventive chemotherapy as a preventive measure. One limitation of this strategy is the inability to prevent re-infection, and infection rates tend to return to baseline within 24 months after the drug therapy. Therefore, the strategy has to be repeated with a frequency befitting the endemicity of schistosomiasis in the area.

The Cyprian Plague

This pestilence was reported first in the city of Alexandria in 249 AD. It was with the troops that the soldiers spread it to one another. It was then reported in Rome in the following year. It rapidly spread to Greece, Rome, and Syria. This plague had devastating effects on the globe because it happened 70 years after the Antonine plague, and people had not fully recovered from it. This plague was named the Cyprian Plague after, Saint Cyprian, the bishop of Carthage. He not only observed and documented signs and symptoms but also the progress of the disease. He also urged Christians to be compassionate to the sick and dying. This was the key to survival during this great pestilence. Being a bishop and not a medical person, Cyprian gives a very interesting perspective in the understanding of the disease. This plague scourged the people and caused immense corporal suffering. This suggests that the people did not have immunity against this plague as they had not encountered it before. The plague caused huge suffering among the people, physical, emotional as well as mental suffering. Cyprian suggested that it was the end of the world. It spread so rapidly due to warfare that was occurring at that time. For instance, the Roman Empire was enduring attacks from German tribes at Gaul and by the Parthians in Mesopotamia. During the war, the soldiers came in contact with each other, rapidly spreading the disease. The disease was spread by airborne droplets, and contact with the infected persons. The disease was also spread indirectly via contaminated clothes and utensils. Contact with infected corpses also spread the plague, and for this reason, the people treated the corpse and disposed of it as fast as they could. Cyprian recorded the symptoms of the plague based on first-hand observations. Since he suffered from this disease, we can confidently say that we are learning from the horse's mouth. In his book De Mortalite, he explained that the sufferers of the disease experienced bouts of diarrhea. In his words, their bowels got loose, and the stool was bloody. The patients would also vomit continuously. This, combined with diarrhea, caused the patients to be very dehydrated.

Unlike the previous pandemics, the plague caused deafness and blindness. Their legs and feet became paralyzed, and this suggested that the nervous system was affected. The patients experienced excruciating pain and delirium. Modern scientists suggest that the plague could have been comprised of Meningitis and another disease. Cyprian also documents that the patients also had blood in the eyes, which is also known as conjunctival bleeding. Their mouths were stained, and their throats were sore. This was due to the inflammation of the mucosal membranes of the mouth and esophagus. The patients would cough unceasingly, and they, therefore, had difficulty while swallowing their food. In severe cases, the contagion caused falling off of the extremities of the limbs. The plague eventually caused the painful death of the patients. Historians and scientists speculate that the plague could have been bubonic plague, smallpox virus, typhus, anthrax or Ebola. Scientists ruled out bubonic plague due to the lack of mention of buboes. Smallpox was definitely not the disease because the witnesses had no account of full-body rash. The most accurate speculation is that the pestilence was a combination of Ebola-due to the bleeding and necrosis, Meningitis-due to the impact on the nervous system and swollen feet and Acute Bacillary Dysentery which is characterized by continuous diarrhea. They also concluded that this disease was one of the first cases of zoonotic diseases. They believe that it was transferred from animals to man. This explains the viciousness of the symptoms and the high death toll. The disease did not come to an abrupt end but had seasonality. It recurred mostly during winter, in the course of the plague. During the 3rd Century, knowledge in medicine was sparse. The people thought that the plague was a punishment from God. Cyprian explains that the pagans thought that the existence of the Christian religion caused the gods to burn with rage, and for this, they scourged the earth with the pestilence. They also held that the drought, famine, and at times, floods that had happened before the plague was due to this reason. Both the Christians and pagans held that the disease was caused by supernatural forces, only that Christians saw it as a test for their faith, rather than a punishment. Christians also believed that the world was coming to an end. They held the belief that the disease was a part of the process of the apocalypse. They had faith that those who would endure this 'temptation' would have a better after-life. The plague spread far and wide. From Alexandria, it spread quickly to other coastal towns. It spread to all areas, rural and urban. The people thought that the disease was spread by corrupted air that was spreading throughout the empire. The Athenians believed that the disease was transmitted through the clothes. The speed at which the disease spread convinced the people that the disease could be transmitted just by sight. This was further fortified by the fact that the disease caused the conjunctival hemorrhage. The fact that the disease affected the eyes caused it to be dreaded far and wide. The people held the eyes as special organs which had tactile energy. They believed that the eyes of the victims of the disease could reach out and touch, thus transmitting the disease. The plague provided an opportunity for the immense growth of Christianity. The Christians tried to explain the propagation of the disease and measures that the people could take to avoid catching it. Cyprian told the people at Carthage that the plague, which seemed horrible, was an opportunity to love the sick and to take care of them. He urged the Christians to take care of the sick, kinsmen, or not, selflessly. As the disease was highly contagious, some contracted it in the process. When they died, it was assumed to be martyrdom. The pagans, on the other hand, did nothing or very little to try and combat the spread of the disease. They fled from their friends in an attempt to avoid contracting the disease. As imagined, the people lost faith in paganism and started practicing Christianity. Dionysius, the Bishop of Alexandria, reported that the Christians took care of the sick regardless of the danger. The heathen, he said, fled the sick and dying, regardless of the previous relationship with them. This was a period in which the people felt utterly helpless. Cyprian said that the plague intensified the sense of morality and fragility. The Christians urged the people to spend their precious moments of life following the pearls of wisdom and teachings of Christ Jesus. The Cyprian plague took many souls. It is estimated that each day 5,000 people died. It affected all, both young and old. In total, it claimed 60-70 million lives. This was much higher than the death toll during the Antonine Plague. People were in great pain. The plague caused so many deaths that even the rites of death were no longer observed. In the funerary complex of Harwa and Akhi Menu, some of the victims of the Cyprian Plague were buried. Modern scientists speculate that the bodies were disposed hastily according to the arrangements of the corpses. The bodies were covered in a thick layer of lime. It was historically used as a disinfectant. Scientists attempted to extract the DNA of the contagion from human remains. However, the climate of Egypt caused the disintegration and complete destruction of the DNA, making it very difficult to pin-point the contagion. The workforce in the fields was greatly diminished, and agriculture was drastically affected. The collapse of agricultural productivity rendered some lands useless, and some turned into swamps. This led to a famine that affected the people. The lack of food meant that the immunity of people was low, and their bodies could barely fight the plague. The military forces lacked enough soldiers and other military personnel, such as cooks and designers of various types of armor. The disease affected all, regardless of the class in society, gender, age, or religion. In the Roman Empire, two emperors died in the course of the 20 years that this pestilence prevailed. They were Hostilian, in 251 AD, and Claudius Gothicus, in 270 AD. This caused chaos due to political instability in the empire. The leaders who were in place were trying to take the throne; hence the Romans lacked a guardian during this crisis. In conjunction with bad leadership, the diminishing number of soldiers led to the enfeebling of the Roman Army. Rome was in peril of external attacks, and when that happened, she was unshielded. This is one of the reasons why the 3rd Century is considered one of the darkest times in the history of Rome. It almost led to the collapse of the empire. The plague caused people to flee from the cities and towns they lived in. These places were unsanitary as well as crowded. This may explain why the city-dwellers contracted the plague more easily. Some of them were abandoned for good. The bishop of Alexandria explains that the city lost so many people, young and old. The population of the city declined by about 62% from about 500,000 to 190,000 people. He, however, admitted that the decline was not only caused by the deaths caused by the disease, but also the multitude that fled in fear of contracting the disease. The human race was wasted by the desolation of the pestilence. The plague devastated the economy in several ways. The collapse of agricultural production not only caused famine but also cut off some commodities of the trade such as beverages, cotton, and foodstuff. Trade dwindled during the plague due to the reduced number of traders, and meager quantities of goods at a very dear price in the market meant that only a few people could afford them. Taxpayers were not only sick but also economically drained due to the resources they were using to take care of the patients. The Christian community was part of the society that was least affected by the plague. They came up with suggestions to slow the spread of the plague. The few of them who were affected were well taken care of by their brothers and sisters who knew not abandoning. At the peak of despair and turmoil, they were calm and full of hope. They were looking forward to a life after death. Their religion preached endurance during hardship, and this rendered them the resilience of a rock. In following the examples of Jesus, they were compassionate to the ailing pagans and gave them hope of something better than mortality. This moved the pagans, healthy and ailing alike, making them convert into Christianity. At the end of the plague, the church had not only grown in number but also faith and endurance. The Cyprian Plague is arguably the most intriguing pestilence in history. One of the reasons is because its cause has not been well established up to date. It is a plague that taught human beings the importance of supporting each other during crises. It brings out the fragility of the human race in the face of an unseen microbial enemy. It shows how pandemics can wreak havoc and cause people to abandon their normal way of life. The Cyprian Plague shows the gravity of crises as they can shift power economically or politically. The plague also shows that panic plays no part in the solving of crises but only worsens them. It also highlights the effects of a pandemic on the social lifestyle of human beings.

Leprosy

Leprosy is an age-old infectious disease caused by bacillus *Mycobacterium leprae*. The causative organism mainly infects the skin as it majorly thrives in temperatures lower than those within the human body. It has a relatively long incubation period that ranges from one to five years. This is due to the 13-day doubling time of the pathogen. There is a notable tendency of the mycobacterium to invade the nerve cells giving the disease its clinical feature of numbness over the affected area of the body. Besides humans, another documented reservoir of the infective organism is the armadillo. This host is preferred due to its lower body temperature, which favors the proliferation and multiplication of *mycobacterium leprae*. Since ancient civilizations, leprosy has been documented to affect and inflict pain on humans. The earliest possible documentation that many scholars account to be the disease is the Egyptian Papyrus document dating back to around 1550 B.C. Around 600 B.C Indian writings describe an infection that, unanimously, scholars have equated its description to leprosy. In Europe, the first cases of leprosy were recorded in ancient Greece during Alexander's reign. This occurred after his troops returned from India. This coincided with the reported incidences in Rome around 62 B.C., concurrently occurring with the return of Pompeii's troops from Asia Minor. This specifically depicted the presence of the disease in Asia and India. There are other documented cases of the disease seen among the Jews in their ancient writings by their prophets and leaders. Some can be read in the Bible as the phrase "leprosy" is used close to seventy times in the Bible. This term has been used in the Old Testament to refer to an infectious disease affecting the skin. The way the affected patients were handled through isolation and quarantine given to them reflects how highly contagious the disease might have been then. There's no doubt that the same has been observed in recent times concerning handling of the cases of the disease. Jesus is documented healing a man with leprosy in the New Testament. Though these cases cannot be scientifically proven and accurately dated back, their documentation in such a widely read and believed book by a huge part of the world's population is of some significance in understanding that leprosy has affected humans for a long period. Throughout its history, leprosy has been dreaded and misunderstood by the greater part of the population. For long before documentation of its cause, it was thought to be a hereditary infection, a curse, or a punishment from God for the evils done. The infected persons were handled with a lot of stigmas. They were shunned from the rest of the community and left to suffer the infliction solely. During the Middle Ages in Europe, leprosy patients were required to wear certain types of clothing and even bells that would warn the rest of the people of their presence for them to be avoided. Different paths were isolated to be taken by these patients different from those of the healthy population. The direction of wind determined the movements taken in these paths. In the recent past, nothing was much different as the same was done. The infected were left to live in colonies called leprosarium. The presence of this disease impacted the social and cultural ways of human beings. In some ancient communities, there were some forms of artwork done to depict the appearance of leprosy patients. It depicted the scarred and ugly skin characterized by sores on the affected parts. The current history of leprosy is documented from the discovery of the causative microbe in 1873 by Dr. Gerhard Henrik Hansen. This marked the beginning of a series of experimental and clinical interventions developed to treat the sick. Early in the 20th century, doctors treated patients by injecting them with oil from chaulmoogra nut. There were significant cases of recovery though the injection was severely painful. Furthermore, long-term use of such a mode of treatment was questionable. In 1921, the US created a research and treatment center in Carville. This led to a tremendous milestone made in the management of leprosy cases. Development of a sulfone drug called Promin to manage leprosy infections was successful though the injections to be taken were many and painful. In the 1950s, Dapsones pills were discovered in the same research center. This became the drug of choice in treating leprosy; however, *mycobacterium leprae* developed resistance to dapsone. This necessitated the development of multidrug treatment of leprosy in the 1970s. The World Health Organization then recommended the use of this technique to curb these infections. Currently, the same multidrug regimen stands to be used to cure the disease. It contains a combination of Dapsone, Rifampicin, and Clofazimine. This has greatly aided in preventing the development of drug resistance. A 6-month or more course of the drugs is adequate to cure leprosy depending on its severity. Scientists are working tirelessly to come up with a vaccine to help prevent the disease and even to come up with means of detecting the disease early enough before it becomes severe or clinically depicted. Leprosy is thought to be spread from human to human through respiratory droplets or nasal discharges from an infected person when one coughs. Though its incidence currently is rare, in endemic areas, contact with the infected persons could lead to one contracting the disease. Other means of infection include contact with the vectors such as insects or infected soil. It is important to note that currently, most people have conferred a strong immunity to *mycobacterium leprae*. Therefore, most of the people that could be hosts of the pathogen have no clinical presentations of the disease. Clinical presentation of leprosy notably comes late, following the infection with the pathogen. This, as stated earlier, is due to the long incubation period ranging from five to several years of the sub-clinical disease. Moreover, with clinical cases, they vary depending on the severity of the disease. There are two clinical forms of the disease. These are the paucibacillary and multibacillary leprosy. Paucibacillary is a milder form of the disease, while multibacillary is severe. The disease mainly presents with cutaneous areas of hypopigmentation characterized by thickened peripheral nerves. These lesions have numbness with loss of sensation to touch, extremes of cold and heat, pain, and deep pressure depending on its severity. The feet and hands are the body parts commonly affected. In severe lepromatous cases, the involvement of the eyes is seen. In such cases, the eyes could have glaucoma, increased intraocular pressure, loss of visual acuity, or in worse cases, blindness. The involvement of nasal mucosa is seen in multibacillary forms with cases of nasal congestion and epistaxis. Leprosy diagnosis is clinical. This involves the presence of the cardinal signs of areas of hypopigmentation, thickened peripheral numbness, and the presence of numbness over the area in question. A positive slit-skin smear is a confirmation test for the infection. It's prudent to note that diagnosis is an area of interest as research is ongoing to come up with better ways of detecting the disease early in its subclinical stages. This will help reduce cases of human-human infection. For the past twenty years, there has been a decline in the newly recorded cases of leprosy infections annually. In 2001, there were 775,000 new cases. This had notably declined compared to 1988 when WHO identified 122 countries as hot-bed areas for the disease. In 2002, elimination was noted in most of the endemic areas previously identified. This was in exception of 14 countries that still had a prevalence of more than 1 for every 10,000 people. The positive decline in cases in the other 108 countries can be attributed to the widespread use and campaign for the use of multidrug regimens in managing active infections. Currently, there are countries identified as still areas of the prevalence of the disease. These are India, Mozambique, Myanmar, Nepal, and Madagascar. India remains the country with the highest prevalence. This can be attributed to its high population. Cumulatively, the South East Asia region becomes the area with a higher prevalence of leprosy as compared to Africa and America. The epidemiological situation, as per 2015, reported a decline in new cases from 2001 to 211,973 new cases. This showed a tremendous improvement in trying to decrease the number of new cases. However, 94 percent of the reported cases were from 14 countries and the remaining 6 percent from the rest of the world. Areas of high endemicity remain high. Therefore, an effort has to be made to reduce, if not eliminate, the occurrence of new cases. This can be easily achieved by the detection of all the active clinical and subclinical cases and providing adequate treatment of the same. Over the past 20 years, close to twenty million patients have been cured of leprosy using multidrug therapy. This is a great milestone in the fight against leprosy. In 2016, WHO launched a plan to help eradicate leprosy from the world population and the endemic areas. This termed as the Global Leprosy Strategy 2016-2020, was a well-outlined plan founded on three pillars. The pillars entailed the need to stop leprosy and its complications, to stop discrimination and promote inclusion of the affected patients, and finally to strengthen various governments and enable them to participate actively in the eradication of the burden of leprosy. With the mission of promoting a leprosy free world, a focus had to be made on children and to avoid the occurrence of disabilities in case of the disease. Various measures were put in place to aid in this prudent strategy. These include the provision of resources to the affected states, creating community awareness of the disease through campaigns, and creating an e-health network to provide information on the offending disease. Recent interventions to curb leprosy are all based on the Global Leprosy Strategy. In this plan, it is important to note the key measures applied. Researches and establishment of partnerships form the cornerstone of this strategy. It was agreed that there should be a timely detection of new cases and to make sure that all patients on multidrug therapy complete their full course to evade the possible development of drug resistance. The period of drug intake is to vary depending on the kind of disease that one has. For paucibacillary leprosy, a 9-month drug course of PB-MDT has to be completed within 12 months, and in cases of multibacillary leprosy, a 12-month drug dose of MB-MDT has to be completed within 18 months. A follow-up should be made to ensure the completion of the drug therapy and a report to follow the same. BCG vaccine was to be administered to aid in disease prevention. Moreover, a drug supply database should be created to monitor delivery to the affected region. All these, among others, are the current stipulations to achieve the mission of the 2016-2020 strategy. What is the impact of leprosy on an individual's quality of life? Leprosy, if left untreated, may lead to progressive physical, psychological, and social disabilities. Often, this is as a result of the stigma that these patients have to cope with from the community in which they are brought up. This depicts the kind of misery, and mental torture one undergoes in cases where there's a confirmed case. The poor health-seeking behavior in most of the suspected cases can be attributed to the fear of isolation from friends and even in worst cases, family. In countries such as India and Myanmar, where the prevalence of leprosy is relatively high, the infected cannot freely visit places of worship as there is a fear of cross-infection on healthy persons. Due to the delayed health-seeking behavior, most patients end up with physical disabilities that can only be corrected at an expensive cost, even post healing of leprosy. Many such patients cannot afford reconstructive surgery to eliminate the scarred skin, hypopigmented lesions, or even correct the eye lesions, that at worse, could lead to irreversible blindness. Thus, it is important to note that leprosy is documented as a communicable disease with higher incidences of permanent physical disability as a consequence. In conclusion, leprosy is a disease that has been around since ancient civilizations presenting to be highly infectious. Knowledge of its causation marked a change in the way the affected persons were viewed. The notion of it being a curse or having familial delineation was abolished. Advancements in its management have been noted with a tremendous decrease in its prevalence within the past two decades. WHO has outlined a strategy aimed at eradicating the disease and preventing any further new cases in the whole world. This is guiding current interventions to curb the disease. Therefore, with strict follow up on the stated strategy, new cases of leprosy are to be avoided, and the confirmed should be healed with decreased chances of developing disabilities among the infected through early detection of disease.

Conclusion

Man has been facing diseases since time immemorial. It has been nature's way of selecting those who are the fittest to survive. Based on evolution, diseases are a way of eliminating the weaker species which could not fight it. Pandemics have wreaked havoc and planted seeds of uncertainty in people's lives. Most have caused millions of deaths, while others have left behind victims who are crippled for life. Some diseases have left people with a stronger resolve to survive, while other pandemics highlight the fragility and mortality of human beings. More often than not, we tend to see just the effects on the people's health and the society's health system, but we overlook other significant outcomes that pandemics have. The pandemics and epidemics impact the social lives of victims immensely. The relationships with each other have either been fortified or torn down to pieces. The blame-game that comes along with crises leaves many relationships shattered beyond repair. On the other hand, those that unite together to fight the crisis have always had stronger and better relationships. Some religions have grown immensely thanks to the pandemics, which to them, are a blessing in disguise. For instance, during the Plague of Cyprian, Christianity grew immensely due to the increased number of followers who felt a sense of hope in the faith. Other religions lost meaning because they did not offer enough explanation for the trouble the people encountered. Pandemics have a way of disrupting the fabric of society. At times the fabric becomes tighter, and at others, it falls apart, losing its meaning. Pandemics can cause the upholding of morals or the shunning of the same. The plague of Athens saw disorder infiltrate the lives of the inhabitants of the city. The laws of man or God were not heeded, and this was a period of utter dysfunction and chaos. The HIV/AIDS pandemic, on the other hand, made a great deal of the population improve on sexual immorality in a significant way. Each disease, in its own little way, changes society. The Japan smallpox pandemic, which mainly affected small children, made them valuable and cherishable so that the 'smallpox demon' could not reap their souls. Disease affects the political standing of a nation. Whether it is the politics of a particular country or a region, pandemics have not shunned from disrupting the politics when the opportunity arises. The pestilences caused the demise of leaders. Marcus Aurelius, a remarkable leader, died during the Antonine Plague. His death was a massive blow to the city of Rome, which was at war at that time. The citizens also became very demoralized because he was a source of inspiration to many. His son, Commodus, has been said to have contributed to the fall of the Roman Empire. In the olden days, when plagues occurred, they affected the military, weakening their position in battle. The unaffected armies took advantage of the situation and brought down the plagued troops. This way, some nations, and empires lost part of their territories for a while or forever changing the history of our planet. Thus were born new populations and nations that changed the world of their ancestors. In this way, these new generations have laid the foundations for the future to the present day. What we are is also the result of this natural and social selection process. Modern technology will certainly influence more than in the past but Mother Nature has always shown us that in the end, the last word is always hers.

I hope you enjoyed this book! If you like, leave a positive review with your impressions on the Amazon page. I would be really grateful! Check my other books in the Author Page on Amazon, you will find them very interesting! See you at the next reading!

For any kind of request, clarification or advice, feel completely free to contact me at the following email address: davidanversa.author@gmail.com
Thank you very much
David Anversa

Printed in Great Britain
by Amazon